W0112983

"In the rush of modern psychology to find acceptance among the empirical sciences which dominated the last two centuries, mainstream psychology forgot the core of what it means to be human: the need for meaning, and the various pathologies which arise out of the thwarting of spiritual life. The authors of this study called *Principles of InnerView Guidance* seek to reconnect the life of the spirit with the disorders of mind and body, and as such, bring a powerful summons for inclusion of the reality of the soul in the work of healing." – James Hollis

> **Dr. James Hollis** is a Jungian analyst in Washington, DC and author of 16 books, the latest being *Living Between Worlds: Finding Personal Resilience in Changing Times*.

"It is refreshing and heartening to read the ways in which the authors champion the perspective of the soul rather than that of the ego. I heartily recommend this book to all who are concerned with the inner life." – Lionel Corbett

> **Dr. Lionel Corbett** trained in medicine and psychiatry in England and as a Jungian analyst at the C.G. Jung Institute of Chicago. He is the author of *The Sacred Cauldron: Psychotherapy as a Spiritual Practice*.

"*Principles of InnerView Guidance* is an absorbing, intelligent, and most of all, encouraging guide for therapists – and clients on a path to wholeness. Combining an historical perspective with the best contemporary findings, the book forms a bridge between authentic presence and the inner world. In addition, we find a cogent sense of *soul* as deeply significant in therapy and in life. We have seen many books attempting to integrate psychological work and spiritual practice. I see this book as highly successful in that endeavor." – David Richo

> **David Richo** is author of *Triggers: How to Stop Reacting and Start Healing* (Shambhala, 2019).

"In a secular, materialist culture, the irrepressible spiritual dimension of human experience and understanding has been badly neglected for too long. The work of Speyer and Yaphe takes an important step towards correcting that omission. InnerView Guidance, uniquely beneficial in terms of personal growth to both client and healer, may well be the healthiest approach to psychological care yet invented. This fine book, calmly asserting the essential truth that *spiritually whole lives matter*, deserves the widest possible readership. It is a masterpiece of therapeutic wisdom, kindness and care." – Larry Culliford

> **Larry Culliford** is a retired physician and psychiatrist from Sussex, UK. He is the author of several influential books including *The Psychology of Spirituality, Much Ado about Something*, and *The Big Book of Wisdom*. He also posts regularly to a long-running blog for *Psychology Today* under the byline: *Spiritual Wisdom for Secular Times*.

"This book is a scholarly and heartfelt weaving together of the personal, interpersonal, and transpersonal aspects of psychotherapy. InnerView and the 4Fold Path are excellent models for understanding how the sometimes ineffable dimensions of soul and spirit can be practically implemented in clinical practice, for a much richer, deeper, and more profound treatment effect. Designed for professionals, it is also a great read for anyone interested in the depth dimensions of psychology." – Cassandra Vieten

> **Cassandra Vieten** is Visiting Scholar, University of California San Diego, Executive Director, John W. Brick Mental Health Foundation, Senior Fellow and Past President, Institute of Noetic Sciences, and author of *Spiritual and Religious Competencies in Clinical Practice: Guidelines for Psychologists and Mental Health Professionals*.

"There is a fresh and original approach here and though they base their work on preceding theorists in a good way, the book is clearly on the leading edge in its field. I find the scholarship outstanding. The authors' grasp of the history of psychotherapy and of spiritual counselling, and their command of the literature is very reassuring. The book is timely and should become a foundational text with a long life." – Philip McKenna

> **Philip McKenna** is a former Dominican priest and has worked as a psychodynamic psychotherapist in Canada for the last 50 years. He was one of the founders of the Centre for Training in Psychotherapy and a member of the Transitional Council of the College of Registered Psychotherapists of Ontario (CRPO).

"Finally, the best aspects of psychology/spirituality/soul-work have been melded into one modality that can promote healing and thriving instead of focusing primarily on pathology. There is a current wave of new findings in neuropsychology and epigenetics that is focused on the mind-body-spirit connection. This will be a great fit for the world of psychology to provide a new approach to therapy that complements the new directions of science. I am a practitioner and would have this book on hand for reference and use in clinical work." – Madison L. Akridge

> **Madison L. Akridge** is a licensed clinical social worker and board certified coach. Her background includes a BA in philosophy, master of social work, postgraduate training in applied behavior analysis, EMDR, Heart-Centered Hypnotherapy®, comprehensive energy psychology, and integrative wellness/life coaching.

Applications of a Psychospiritual Model in the Helping Professions

This book brings together the historically separate domains of mental health and spiritual awareness in a holistic framework called InnerView Guidance. Building on strength-based and solution-oriented approaches to therapy, the InnerView model offers a unique psychospiritual approach which can be applied in any of the helping professions.

InnerView recognizes the individual's need for internal cohesion between psychological growth and spiritual development. It is a principle-driven paradigm that foregrounds 'soul work' as a central evolutionary task. The book presents the core concepts and methodology involved in the alignment of ego with soul. Chapters explain the theoretical roots of the model, explore practical applications in therapeutic settings, and introduce InnerView as a rich synergy of psychotherapy and spiritual guidance.

Taking an original and cutting-edge approach, this valuable text will be essential reading for scholars and students, as well as practitioners in the fields of psychotherapy, counselling, life coaching, social work, and spiritual care.

Cedric Speyer is a writer and Registered Psychotherapist (RP) based in Canada. He is Director of InnerView Guidance International (IGI).

John Yaphe is a family physician with a special interest in counselling. He is Associate Professor at the School of Medicine of the University of Minho, Portugal.

Explorations in Mental Health

For more information about this series, please visit: www.routledge.com/
Explorations-in-Mental-Health/book-series/EXMH

Applications of a Psychospiritual Model in the Helping Professions

Principles of InnerView Guidance

Cedric Speyer and John Yaphe

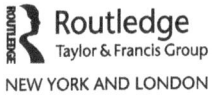

Routledge
Taylor & Francis Group

NEW YORK AND LONDON

First published 2021
by Routledge
52 Vanderbilt Avenue, New York, NY 10017

and by Routledge
2 Park Square, Milton Park, Abingdon, Oxon, OX14 4RN

Routledge is an imprint of the Taylor & Francis Group, an informa business

Library of Congress Cataloging-in-Publication Data
Names: Speyer, Cedric, author. | Yaphe, John, author.
Title: The applications of a psychospiritual model in the helping
    professions : principles of innerview guidance / Cedric Speyer, John Yaphe.
Description: New York, NY : Routledge, 2021. | Series: Explorations in
    mental health | Includes bibliographical references and index.
Identifiers: LCCN 2020033983 (print) | LCCN 2020033984 (ebook) |
    ISBN 9780367894351 (hardback) | ISBN 9781003019152 (ebook)
Subjects: LCSH: Mental illness—Alternative treatment. | Psychotherapy—
    Religious aspects. | Psychiatry and religion.
Classification: LCC RC489.S676 S63 2020 (print) | LCC RC489.S676
    (ebook) | DDC 616.89/14—dc23
LC record available at https://lccn.loc.gov/2020033983
LC ebook record available at https://lccn.loc.gov/2020033984

ISBN: 978-0-367-89435-1 (hbk)
ISBN: 978-1-003-01915-2 (ebk)

Typeset in Bembo
by Apex CoVantage, LLC

To Tom Francoeur. Your self-giving continues through our work.

For Maurice, Elizabeth, and Geoffrey Speyer, and Maria Eusebia da Silva.

With love to Ze, Ju, and Anna and in memory of Wilf, Ruth, and Arona.

Contents

Figures

Acknowledgements

The authors began collaborating at age 12 by surreptitiously passing notes back and forth in class, even after our esteemed elementary school teacher Shulamis Yelin, put more distance between our desks. We are grateful for the passion she instilled in us for literature and the humanities and for the written dialogue we discovered, as progenitors of asynchronous online counselling.

No one creates anything on their own. Even a hermit belongs to the community they stand apart from. We are indebted to the individuals and communities who have nurtured and supported our personal development and accompanied us on our professional path.

Cedric Speyer is grateful to all who have taught him the art of Inner-View, from Rustaan to Marilyn.

John Yaphe would like to acknowledge the influence of Arthur Furst and Michael Weingarten on his professional development and clinical work.

We are indebted to many friends and colleagues who have helped hone the ideas in this book over the years. Eusebia da Silva, DeeAnna Nagel, Scott Christie, and Andrea Bassett, are the team behind us, offering invaluable development, design, and editorial support.

Thank you to Elsbeth Wright, our knowledgeable and dedicated editor at Routledge, who provided guidance and encouragement in every phase of the publishing process. Our thanks also go to Bethany White for her support in seeing the manuscript through to the present edition, as we envisioned it.

Finally, to our families and friends, who have put up with long editorial meetings and writing sessions while this book was a work in progress, thank you for being there.

We are grateful to the many people we have had the privilege to know along the way, who have taught us what soul work involves, far beyond what we have learned from our own reflection and introspection. It is a blessing to have such travelling companions on the evolutionary journey.

Foreword

Michael Delmonte

This is a timely yet forward-thinking book which seeks to restore soul work from the wisdom traditions to modern therapeutic practice. To this end, the authors present the synthesis of clinical and spiritual approaches they call InnerView. The integration of the empirical legacy of psychology with the heritage of soul-centred wisdom is not new. Much has been said and written about the need to revitalize a field in which the whole person is often compartmentalized into brain functions and behavioural mechanisms in the name of scientific objectivity. The contribution of this book clearly comes from the holistic camp. Yet it travels further along the road less travelled. It puts psychospiritual theory into practice based on the founding principles of InnerView clinical philosophy as delineated in each of the chapters. Those principles, which have successfully guided countless coaching, counselling, and therapy sessions, have now been brought into clear view for professional helpers from various domains, who have much to gain from learning the soul psychology introduced here. By emphasizing "what the soul wants" in the therapeutic encounter, the authors bring a refreshing perspective to the consultation room. They have literally mapped out an overview of personhood (the 4Fold Path map of Chapter 4) beyond that of personality theories. In so doing, readers are offered a new vision of psychospiritual realities beyond those associated with the self-imposed limits of traditional clinical psychology.

Reality is complex. It can be experienced across a wide spectrum of levels, from the very concrete to difficult-to-pin-down abstractions. At the concrete level we have the physical reality of the natural world around us, including various life-forms such as plants, animals, and human beings. At the intermediate level there is the psychosocial domain of human interactions, experienced in the culturally specific expressions of language, dress codes, statues, flags, music, painting, architecture, and so forth. At the most abstract level we surmise the existence of a spiritual domain reflected in the many great wisdom traditions. In the age-old evolution of spiritual wisdom, Sikhism and Buddhism emerged from Hinduism, with Christianity and Islam rooted in Judaism. In the Far East, the refinements of spiritual seeking are evident in Taoism and Confucianism in China, and Shintoism in Japan. A cursory survey like this underscores that there is a wealth of psychospiritual development throughout human history that can only serve to enrich psychology without having to abandon its secular advances.

Most healing traditions have focused on the concrete end of the spectrum as is the case with physical medicine. The long and noble tradition of medicine goes back to the ancient Greeks in the West, and to Egyptian, Indian, and Chinese medicine in the East. The Eastern traditions tend to be holistic in their approach to health, with body, mind, and spirit considered unified with respect to well-being. However, in the West, medicine has become increasingly fractured into specialties. This approach tends to treat the human body parts in a disparate way; it tends to separate the mind from the body and both from the spirit, while relegating the latter to the religious sphere, not considered the professional business of doctors.

Thankfully, about a century ago physicians such as Sigmund Freud, Carl Jung, and Alfred Adler brought the mind and deeper psyche back into the picture. They paid attention to the subjective experience of patients as a reality of assessment. Whereas Freud delved into childhood trauma for the sources of mental illness, Adler emphasized the challenges that the tasks of life presented in the psychosocial domain. Jung, however, was more interested in the underlying collective archetypes making life profoundly meaningful. In other words, Jung brought the spiritual domain into psychological view. He was followed in this endeavour by others such as Viktor Frankl, Erich Fromm, and Rollo May. However, spiritual considerations in the helping professions have largely been neglected, being difficult to measure and test scientifically. Hence the timely value of this lucid contribution by Cedric Speyer and John Yaphe.

This groundbreaking book builds on the strong foundations of humanistic and positive psychology. One can also discern the influence of Jungian thought in the book, as well as that of Hegelian dialectics, existential psychology, and Celtic spirituality from the West. A well-informed background in both Western and Eastern philosophical traditions is evident, the latter especially related to meditation and mindfulness-based practices. The comprehensive spiritual perspective is brought down to earth by the authors' inclusive knowledge of psychodynamic therapy, behaviour therapy, cognitive therapy, narrative therapy, coaching, and solution-focused therapy. All in all, although the authors reach for the sky, their feet are firmly on the ground! Many people search for meaning in their lives – not just pills and cognitive-behavioural fixes to relieve depression and anxiety. However, the authors understand the need for a secure psychological base to facilitate soul work. Ultimately, the striving ego is not meant to be our master. The ego is at its best when it serves the "bigger story" of human evolution in which we are all immersed.

Dr. Michael (Michelo) Delmonte was born in The Hague and educated in Dublin. He holds primary degrees in genetics and psychology, as well as a higher diploma in education, a research MSc, and a PhD in psychology. He obtained an MPsychSc in psychotherapy from University College, Dublin, and conducted psychotherapy at St. James's Hospital, St. Patrick's University Hospital, and St. Edmundsbury Hospital, where he was Principal Psychologist. Currently in private practice, he lectures at both Trinity College and University College, Dublin. Dr. Delmonte has published more than 90 articles on psychotherapy, meditation, mindfulness, and evolution. He is the author, with Maeve Halpin, of *Evolution and Consciousness: From a Barren Rocky Earth to Artists, Philosophers, Meditators and Psychotherapists*, published in 2019 by Brill/Rodopi.

Preface

Cedric Speyer

> If we treat people as they are, we make them worse. If we treat people as what
> they could be, we help them become what they are capable of becoming.
> – Johann Wolfgang von Goethe

This book presenting the basic principles of the InnerView model has
been two years in the making, yet its origins go back much further. My
coauthor and I were pioneers in the practice of online counselling for
16 years, developing effective methods along the way. Our present theoretical orientation emerged from the primary process with clients and the
feedback we received from them. We went on to apply the best practices
we discovered to the training and supervision of helping professionals in
other domains, as well as to the teaching of medical students. Yet the ideas
informing InnerView Guidance are not just the result of our respective
clinical careers. Without the essential legacies of both psychology and
spirituality, we would not be positioned to explore the synthesis of those
inheritances in the form of soul work. We are grateful for all who came
before us who are precursors of our endeavours.

In the movie *Man of La Mancha*, based on the classic novel *Don Quixote* by Cervantes, there is a woman at the local inn named Aldonza who
considers Don Quixote delusional and offensive when he envisions her as
his virtuous noble lady, Dulcinea. Yet by the end of the film when Don
Quixote is on his deathbed, she comes to him redeemed by his vision of
her. After he dies, when his squire Sancho Panza calls her Aldonza, she
replies, "My name is Dulcinea!" She has become what he loved and loves
the name that called her to become it.

The quote by Goethe at the beginning of this preface encapsulates the
InnerView approach. In the words of a statement attributed to Nelson
Mandela, "It never hurts to think too highly of a person; often they
become ennobled and act better because of it." There is nothing Aldonza

knows of herself that makes her Dulcinea except for how Don Quixote initially relates to her. When it comes to our own potential, all it takes is one person who can see that promise as a present reality, albeit one which has yet to fully manifest. We need someone who sees us in the same way they can envision the butterfly yet to emerge from the cocoon, the oak contained in the acorn, or the seed of a life's purpose before it fully blossoms. I was blessed with such a mentor who related to me as if I already was what I potentially could be long before I was able to live out what he saw in me. This book is one way of paying forward the gift of his guiding vision and wisdom.

Dr. Thomas A. Francoeur (1921–2014) was the 'godfather' of the InnerView model, and I learned the approach from him before we gave it a name. He was my counselling professor, mentor, and spiritual director when my career path was anything but clear to me. After he retired, Dr. Francoeur was Professor Emeritus of the Department of Integrated Studies in Education, McGill University, having taught both counselling psychology and "the psychology of religious response." He kept his office at McGill and continued to see those he counselled starting at seven in the morning and continuing throughout the day, on a pro-bono basis. His genius was seeing people through their emotional and mental issues, without ever perceiving them through the filter of the condition or illness which brought them to him in the first place. That had a profound life-changing effect on those who were referred to him or otherwise sought him out. Throughout his career, many so-called 'hopeless cases' were sent his way and found a profound acceptance they had never before experienced.

In short, Francoeur was a master of attunement (Chapter 6). I had some firsthand experience of practising attunement before becoming a psychotherapist myself. When I worked as a psychiatric attendant, it allowed me to relate to patients without the inherent power-differential of clinician-patient. I had observed that when 'mental patients' were faced with those officially treating them, it reinforced their mental patient status. To be a mental patient you must have a mental illness. In my nonclinical role, the often rigid, fear-based boundary between mental health providers and mentally ill patients could dissolve in an atmosphere of mutual acceptance, behind the veil of roles. It is as if I would say to them, "Okay, you are in this 'condition' and I am in mine. So here we are. What now?"

It was in the psychiatric milieu that I first practised the InnerView principle of meeting behind-the-scenes of problem-saturated stories and disturbed personalities. Later, it was applied to clinical casework. Of course, it was never easy, and far from a cure-all, mainly because on the psychiatric wards, I was not trying to cure anything. However, I noticed how patients responded. In fact, I developed a reputation for being able to calm down psychotic and potentially violent patients, even when they had to be physically restrained. It is an approach we hope to bring to police departments through InnerView trainings.

During this period, in Francoeur's presence and with his guidance, I learned to keep my heart open in the face of pain – both my own and that projected my way. In doing so, I discovered a way of being attentive to the reality of persons beyond the twists and turns of their personalities or life situations. My work in psychiatry exposed me to those who had few social masks left to protect, no normal or tactful filters on the use of language, and relatively little identification with ego status (all stripped away by having landed on one of the bottom rungs of society). That often left them available for direct soul contact, and all one had to do in turn was to be equally accessible on that level. These authentic encounters became part of the inspiration for the InnerView clinical philosophy, which emerged many years later.

When we say that someone has a lot of 'soul', that is the resonance we feel between inner qualities and the outer expression of them. Soul work is the process of narrowing the gap. The InnerView path is about what it takes to stay on the growing edge of soul making. On that quest we need to see with the heart and seek with the soul. It can be a quick study or a long journey because the nature of any psychospiritual growth is to be continuously unfolding. When I told a client outright, "You may have this problem, but the problem does not have you", that was a breakthrough. From then on, case management became more about the client's soul work than their clinical condition. The paradox is that psychology fulfils its potential when it goes beyond what we know of human persons from psychology alone. This book explores the frontier where the horizons of psychology and spirituality converge.

Introduction

In the early twentieth century, Sigmund Freud anticipated a new profession dedicated to the kind of soul psychology we describe in this book. He seems to have envisioned a psychospiritual approach now emerging in our time, one not defined by the domains of either medicine or religion. He wrote to Oskar Pfister: "I should like to hand it [psychoanalysis] over to a profession which does not yet exist, a profession of lay curers of souls who need not be doctors and should not be priests" (Freud, Freud, Pfister, & Meng, 1963). Freud's hand-off has since been carried forward on different fronts within the helping professions. The authors of this book have accepted the invitation by endeavouring to bring the best of psychology and spirituality into a new synthesis for soul work named InnerView Guidance.

One of the first psychotherapists to differentiate the province of the soul from the study of behaviour related to mental and emotional functioning was the Jungian analyst Evangelos Christou. Christou's life was cut short in a car accident in 1956 at the age of 34. His unfinished manuscript, *The Logos of the Soul*, published posthumously in 1976, laid the foundation for the central premises covered in this book many decades later (Christou, 2007). Christou believed that psychology as a science had become dissociated from the soul's point of view as the unifying principle underlying perceiving, feeling, thinking, and willing. Psychology had therefore lost touch with its own subject. Like Freud, he looked forward to the soul being consciously reinstated in psychotherapy, given its capacity to integrate all the parts of ourselves into a single whole life. InnerView Guidance has inherited that mission, with a path and practice based on discerning "what the soul wants" as the deepest nature of our being, our unique way of belonging to life, and the still, small voice of what matters most to us.

The current era seems ready for the transition. The changes in society's attitudes to psychotherapy can be traced in popular films (Schneider, 1987).

In the classic film-noir *Conflict* from 1945, a psychotherapist describes his work to an interested couple. "A thought can be like a malignant disease that starts to eat away at the willpower. When that happens, it is my job to remove the thought before it can cause destruction. . . . Love and its frustrations is the worst offender." This scene exposes the reductionism, negativity bias, and misapplied science that Christou countered with the preeminence of the soul's viewpoint. That kind of pathologizing has continued in one form or another to this day.

InnerView has emerged in the positive psychology era, one in which practitioners are trained to assess strengths and capabilities rather than being overly focused on damage and deficits. There is an increasing shift of professional attention away from the medical model to motivational approaches, as life coaching gains ground in the mental health marketplace. Those in the field of mental health increasingly realize it needs to live up to its name, rather than being the mental illness field it has historically defaulted to instead. It is part of the pendulum swing away from probing emotional wounds for hidden sources of emotional damage. We now search sources of wholeness, for what is right with people rather than what is wrong with them. It is also part of the shift from an egocentric worldview to the soul-based perspective of a more conscious life journey.

Foundations of InnerView Guidance

What do inspirational stories, whether real-life or fictional, have in common? They point towards what the soul wants and what the spirit knows: that our life circumstances take place in a larger psychospiritual landscape. The InnerView path offers a way to navigate that interior terrain and become an experienced guide for others finding their way. Helping professionals here to learn InnerView principles will be reminded of the original meaning of professional both in theory and practice. A mental health professional is not only a qualified practitioner with a toolkit of effective techniques, but also a healer grounded in a profession of faith. That faith is not to be confused with religious doctrine, though the wisdom found in religious traditions may support it. The therapeutic faith behind the InnerView approach is based on the integrity of persons seeking to become who they were born to be, and the matrix of mercy in which that universal quest is embedded.

The poet e. e. cummings reflected on that quest for true personhood when he wrote, "Almost anybody can learn to think or believe or know, but not a single human being can be taught to feel. Why? Because whenever you think or you believe or you know, you're a lot of other people:

but the moment you feel, you're nobody-but-yourself" (Cummings, 1965). That "nobody-but-yourself" comes from expanding one's range of feeling rather than contracting in response to life's challenges. When we shift our point of view from mental illness to mental health, from pathology to possibility, it is like replacing a microscope with a telescope in our vision of the inner life. Carl Jung spoke of outgrowing problems we face, rather than trying to resolve them directly. He suggested that a broadening of outlook could cause seemingly insoluble issues to lose their urgency and fade in the light of a new level of consciousness (Jung, 1931).

There is another significant perspective informing the InnerView model. It involves a shift in the balance of power between ego and soul. It seeks to balance the wise mind and voice of the soul with the clamouring demands of ego. InnerView guidance helps discern between the two, especially when on the outside we can be waylaid by denial and blame, and on the inside subject to distraction and discouragement. When we clearly see the balance of power between ego and soul in any life situation, the choice each person then makes is a matter of their own act of faith.

The Path and Practice of InnerView

After 40 years of medical and clinical practice, including overseeing 100,000 online cases using the InnerView model of short-term counselling, the authors felt it was time to share this psychospiritual model with a wider audience. As a psychotherapist and clinical supervisor (Cedric Speyer) and family physician (John Yaphe), we developed an approach to psychological healing that goes beyond the standard biomedical and cognitive-behavioural approaches prevalent today. We have published a series of articles on InnerView best practices in peer-reviewed journals and textbook chapters directed to an academic audience. Popular columns and articles presenting our methods have reached a wider readership. We feel it is time to describe the theory and its application in greater depth. This book is intended both for practitioners who would like to learn a more soul-based way of relating to clients and for individuals on a path of becoming more psychologically and spiritually conscious.

There is an increasingly recognized interface between psychotherapy and spiritual guidance. Peter Scazzero has claimed in *Emotionally Healthy Spirituality*, "It's impossible to be spiritually mature while remaining emotionally immature" (Scazzero, 2017). Other authors, such as Larry Culliford in *The Psychology of Spirituality* (Culliford, 2011), Lionel Corbett *in The Sacred Cauldron: Psychotherapy as a Spiritual Practice* (Corbett,

2015), and John Welwood in *Toward a Psychology of Awakening* (Welwood, 2002) provide evidence for the overlap between psychology and religious sensibility. To be an ethically sound counsellor or therapist, it is now necessary to be at least aware, if not fully informed of this interface. Cassandra Vieten and Shelly Scammell outline some of the skills required to function in this way in *Spiritual and Religious Competencies in Clinical Practice: Guidelines for Psychotherapists & Mental Health Professionals* (Vieten & Scammell, 2015).

This book contributes to this crossover by presenting the clinical philosophy and practical applications of InnerView Guidance, covering a different principle in each chapter. The first chapter entitled InnerView Landscapes puts InnerView in the historical perspective of the evolution of therapy over decades and reviews prominent clinical theories in comparison and contrast to how the InnerView model evolved. It describes what InnerView has gained from other therapeutic approaches and how we walk the client through the landscape of their life towards its unconsidered horizons.

The Presenting Person describes methods of assessment used to ascertain where the person finds themselves on their path and envisions where they want to go from there. The person may have a problem, but the problem does not have them. We investigate what is right with the person and hold the vision of their healthiest and preferred state, thereby de-pathologizing the person who is hurting or going through a life transition.

The chapter called Living in a Bigger Story positions the role of the therapist as a guide at the crossroads where different dimensions of life intersect. This approach helps expand the client's sense of identity by evoking the perspective from which problems are situated in the larger context of a client's positive history. We explore the kinds of soul formation emerging from the challenges being experienced. The crossroads is where life's contradictions are acutely felt, and where overarching wisdom is needed to embrace the dichotomies without polarizing them.

The 4Fold Path introduces a map featuring compass points of spirit, soul, ego, and psyche, which frame the illustrative template unfolding in sequential phases of the helping process. A case example demonstrates how the four main elements of InnerView guidance, *witness*, *presence*, *essence*, and *guidance* and the four steps of the overarching CARE model, are applied in short-term work with a client.

In the chapter entitled The Matryoshka Method, we use the image of the nesting Russian dolls to describe how to realign outer personas with the essential needs, values, and intentions of the soul. Understanding how to achieve more congruence between the layers enfolding the innermost doll can help to consolidate therapeutic gains and promote further soul growth.

The sixth chapter, entitled InnerView Attunement, explores how the consciousness of the practitioner 'rubs off' on receptive clients who internalize the quality of rapport felt within sessions. The importance of offering empathy to strengthen the therapeutic alliance has been well-documented. Attunement takes it a step further through energetic synchrony directly affecting the emotional regulation of the client. Advanced skills of dual attention and double awareness are introduced as ways practitioners hold the space for creative tensions until clients learn to do it themselves.

In the seventh chapter, The Principles in Practice, we present the perspective of eight practitioners who have applied InnerView principles in their professional work. They each tell a unique story of their professional development related to the themes of the preceding chapters. We hope this will provide readers with further insight into the InnerView model and its potential for application by a variety of helping professionals.

The conclusion summarizes themes from the previous chapters and presents a unified picture of InnerView, with a vision for a comprehensive soul psychology of the future. Practitioner competencies are reviewed, with respect to the attitude, knowledge, and skills needed to develop psychospiritual expertise. Recommendations for training are provided along with references to relevant literature and other resources. The reader is encouraged to engage in further study, personal exploration, and practice, towards the alignment of personality (ego) with what matters most to a person (soul).

We hope that you, the reader, will find new ways to nourish your own soul growth and foster that of others, and continue the quest we have begun here within your own field of practice. We trust you will find this exploration of the psychospiritual landscape as instructive and transformative as we have.

References

Christou, E. (2007). *The logos of the soul*. Putnam, CT: Spring Publications.

Corbett, L. (2015). *Sacred Cauldron: Psychotherapy as a spiritual practice*. Asheville, NC: Chiron Publications.

Culliford, L. (2011). *The psychology of spirituality: An introduction*. London: Jessica Kingsley Publishers.

Cummings, E. E. (1965). *E.E. Cummings: A miscellany revised*. New York, NY: October House.

Freud, S., Freud, E. L., Pfister, O., & Meng, H. (1963). *Psycho-analysis and faith.* London: Hogarth Press.

Jung, C. G. (1931). *The secret of the golden flower. A Chinese book of life. Translated [into German] and explained by Richard Wilhelm with a European commentary by C.G. Jung, etc. (Translated into English by Cary F. Baynes.).* London: Kegan Paul & Co.

Scazzero, P. (2017). *Emotionally healthy spirituality: It's impossible to be spiritually mature, while remaining emotionally immature.* Grand Rapids, MI: Zondervan.

Schneider, I. (1987). The theory and practice of movie psychiatry. *American Journal of Psychiatry, 144,* 996–1002. https://doi.org/10.1176/ajp.144.8.996.

Vieten, C., & Scammell, S. (2015). *Spiritual and religious competencies in clinical practice: Guidelines for psychotherapists and mental health professionals.* Oakland, CA: New Harbinger Publications, Inc.

Welwood, J. (2002). *Toward a psychology of awakening: Buddhism, psychotherapy, and the path of personal and spiritual transformation.* Boston, MA: Shambhala.

1 InnerView Landscapes

Overview of New Horizons in Psychology

InnerView Guidance evokes a wide-angle view of the landscape of therapeutic theories and situates the model within the context of positive psychology – the study of the strengths and virtues enabling people to thrive. Parker J. Palmer speaks to this perspective when he says: "I was already standing on the ground of my new life, ready to take the next step on my journey, if only I would turn around and see the landscape that lay before me. If we are to live our lives fully and well, we must learn to embrace the opposites, to live in a creative tension between our limits and our potentials" (Palmer, 2000).

Psychology, originally meaning knowledge of the soul, had its roots in philosophy before making its claim as a science and being established as a branch of medicine. InnerView puts the emphasis on mental health, without discounting what has been learned about the causes of mental illness. When it comes to the limits of psychology, "The soul has been given its ears to hear things that mind does not understand" (Rumi & Barks, 2004).

Individually and collectively we are called to align our lives with an expansive, ever-evolving sacred story. When it comes to grappling with ground level issues in the lives of clients, this means we are always looking for the healthy, big picture context in which the presenting problem takes place, that is, the life behind the life situation. This involves a vision of the inclusive self beyond the confines of the problem-saturated story (O'Hanlon, 2003).

InnerView guidance is designed to bring seekers of all kinds into alignment with the best of their human nature. When conducted on a short-term basis, it plants the seeds for long-term soul work. It is a matter of realignment with the feelings, needs, values, and purposes which allow our inner and outer worlds to be congruent. That integral coherency in turn opens our limited personal selves to transpersonal and archetypal realms and we come to see our life situation from the broader, more meaningful perspective known as wisdom.

InnerView is about what kind of person is having the problem, rather than what kind of problem is discouraging the person. InnerView moves away from the medical model of therapy and towards the pilgrimage path of psychospiritual guidance. That is, from what is wrong with people to what is right with persons, from pathology to possibilities, from an ego-based framework to a soul-grounded perspective on helping and healing. When we encourage people to see the bigger picture of their heroic life journey, it helps them to disidentify with the self-concept of being psychologically damaged goods. An expansive vision leaves a person feeling good about themselves and others, much like the redemptive end of a romantic comedy will reframe all the prior crisis points in the plot.

How Prominent Therapeutic Approaches Inform InnerView

Many coaches, counsellors, and therapists say they are eclectic in their approach, which means they draw upon a variety of therapeutic methods or clinical protocols. A protocol-driven model is one that provides specific guidelines and a case management structure to follow. A principle-driven model outlines general principles, which invoke supportive protocols, which in turn guides progress towards client goals (Watts, 2013). The difference between the two is similar to the difference between a belief system (theological premises) and a spiritual practice (meditation).

InnerView Guidance is a principle-driven approach that integrates emotional, mental, and spiritual growth. It offers a psychospiritual perspective informing one's own soul work as well as being a way to help and support others. InnerView also offers protocols for problem resolution, yet these are often derived from other models of therapy and can be practised to the extent they align with personal learning styles and resonate with the positive ways emotional, mental, and spiritual growth take place. The following review of the main models in the field intends to show what InnerView has in common with other therapeutic theories and how it differs from them. There is a measure of truth in all these models. No one has the complete picture of the human person, yet all theorists contribute to it. We have much to gain from understanding other perspectives.

Psychodynamic or Analytic Therapy

The traditional approach is sometimes still called Freudian, after Sigmund Freud, the founder of psychoanalysis. More often it is now known as psychodynamic or analytic therapy and has greatly influenced other schools of personality theory. However, it is less common than it was decades ago before short-term adaptations of it gained ground. There are many post-Freudian derivations of this model. In this approach, problems are framed as internalized conflicts between different parts of the personality (id, ego, and superego or child, adult, and parent). These conflicts are repressed (or pushed out of awareness). Therefore, investigating the past is crucial to understanding present problems. Symptoms reflect ways the subconscious mind protects the conscious one from having to deal with the real problem, originating in childhood. An array of defence mechanisms (e.g., denial, regression, projection, dissociation) serve this psychological subterfuge. Problems are resolved when people discover the true motivations for their emotions and actions, and thereby become more conscious than unconscious of their issues. The greater awareness we have of internal complexes, the more freedom we have from compensating symptoms (Duncan, 2005).

From the InnerView perspective, the psychodynamic approach can be a useful way to differentiate emotional programs from the past that still drive the operating system of the psyche in the present, instead of being guided by intentional, individuated motivations. It can also allow for progressive dismantling of the constructed self that is overly identified with outmoded family dramas, unquestioned social conditioning, and unexamined cultural myths. According to this approach, the authentic person can then emerge and flourish.

However, when intrapsychic malfunctions of mind are understood to rule the rest of the personality, clients tend to view themselves as stuck in the rut of what Freud originally termed the *repetition compulsion* – replaying the same patterns while expecting different results. Neuropsychology research has shown that our brains are wired accordingly, to tell ourselves the same story about life situations and repeat the same coping mechanisms, no matter how dysfunctional. Carl Jung, the Swiss psychiatrist who founded Analytical Psychology posited a different way of changing course.

> All the greatest and most important problems of life are fundamentally insoluble . . . they can never be solved, but only outgrown. This "outgrowth" proves on further investigation to require a new level of consciousness. Some higher or wider interest appears on the horizon and through this broadening of outlook the insoluble problem loses its urgency. It is not solved logically in its own terms but fades when confronted with a new and stronger life urge.
>
> (Lü et al., 1962)

InnerView is about encouraging that life-giving sense of expansion, as a prerequisite to any insights about what has thwarted its full expression.

It starts with a steady gaze on the whole person. We can imagine this by reversing the usual figure-ground perspective. Normally we focus on the main object of perception and not on the field in which it is situated. In traditional therapy, the person's pain is front and centre, thereby taking most of the attention. InnerView guidance emphasizes the positive background and context behind the problematic life situation. Issues in the foreground seem much more painful when fixation on the figure is the only point of view.

Behaviour Therapy

The results-oriented methods of change became popular in reaction to the introspective immersion of psychoanalysis. From the practical stance of behaviour therapy, problems develop when a specific situation becomes associated with distress (as is the case with many phobias). The person has learned to link an intense emotional state with an event, resulting from inadvertent conditioning. Mental health issues can also occur when certain behaviours (e.g., acting out) are followed by consequences (e.g., attention) which reinforce the strength of the problematic behaviour. Again, the behaviour is learned due to the reward or punishment contingencies which surround it. However, if problems are learned that way through such juxtaposition, they can be unlearned the same way. The coping response, like progressive relaxation, then supplants a previously learned reaction, like anxiety, to a challenging situation. Once the adaptive stance is learned, it is practised like a dress rehearsal with increasing exposure to the presenting problem. In this way, the person is reconditioned under similar circumstances to first act and then feel differently (Duncan, 2005).

When it comes to the ways we are hard-wired to repeat conditioned responses, the behavioural approach can help anchor a person in actions that reinforce consciously chosen goals. This approach offers practical ways to break mental and emotional habits that oppose what the soul wants. Yet behavioural freedom from debilitating conditions raises the question of what purpose personal freedom serves. This is where psychospiritual development is differentiated from purely psychological interventions. The former involves liberation from the small self or ego identification and shifts the balance of power to the true self. The ego seeks significance in terms of esteem and approval, belonging in terms of security and affection, and meaning in terms of personal empowerment. All these can be achieved by means of attitudinal adjustments and behavioural modifications. Yet when limited to the needs of the ego, we risk flattening the human landscape to its horizontal dimension alone. We will explore this further in Chapter 4, which presents the 4Fold Path.

The soul seeks its worth in terms of the universal human journey, its belonging in terms of a larger Self, and meaning in terms of its part in the unfolding of a bigger, archetypal story. When the soul gains knowledge, experience, and wisdom, it is in service of self-transcending values intrinsic to its essential nature. InnerView represents a new kind of psychospiritual integration. It goes beyond relief from anxiety and depression or addiction to the expansive awareness and qualities of soul it takes to create new psychological structures overriding dysfunctional ones.

Humanistic Therapy

Coinciding with the rise of the human potential movement and its emphasis on the search for meaning and self-actualization, the humanistic approach became a forerunner of the positive psychology movement. This therapeutic approach had its roots in European existential philosophies. Humanistic adherents do not view people as determined by nature and nurture, or socially conditioned by forces shaping their personalities, however much those influences may lead to emotional symptoms or psychological conflicts. From the humanistic perspective, people have the innate capacity to realize their potential and the inherent freedom to fulfil it. The premise underlying this approach is that the basic goodness of the individual can be trusted. Therefore, the solution to life problems lies within the self, the authentic self whose inner world has built-in integrity and self-healing capacities. Problems arise due to incongruence between the ideal self and the authentic self. The ideal self is the person one feels he or she needs to be or should be. The authentic or true self is who one really is, aside from autobiographical story. The wisdom needed to deal with life's challenges is found within; the therapist simply facilitates tuning into it. Under the gaze of unconditional acceptance, the true nature of a person emerges, without interference from theories superimposed in the name of mental health (Duncan, 2005).

From the InnerView perspective, the humanistic approach focuses on the person behind the problem and underscores that a person's life, or what matters most to them, is not defined by their circumstances. It allows for recalibration of significance and belonging based on what is right with the person, and attunement to them based on what is of deepest personal and transpersonal value. The territory of the psyche is like a vast countryside with a river running through it. The polluting or free flowing of that river is the difference between arid soul states and the fruition of full personhood.

Coaching, counselling, and psychotherapy are all forms of learning to become the best versions of ourselves. The Latin root of the word education means to lead out. It reminds us that while exploring the landscape within, people also need to be led out of themselves, from the fixations of an egoic personal identity that sees the world in terms of subject–object polarities, to a unitive consciousness in which the light and dark aspects of human nature are embraced at the crossroads where they intersect. The paradigm shift is equivalent to realizing the earth revolves around the sun rather than the earth being the centre of the universe. For this personal Copernican revolution to occur, we need a vocabulary for the landscape of the soul, one that facilitates psychospiritual guidance. It is important that the practitioner makes space for emotional states such as loneliness, frustration, sadness, and anger, and attends to what those feelings may reveal about unmet needs. Yet a thorough assessment of the client's preferred state of life engagement is also necessary. For example, what memories invoke the qualities of clarity, courage, joy, compassion, wonder, and lovingkindness? What matters to the client beyond the confines of the presenting issue and related ego motivations: security and survival, esteem and affection, and power and control? When we are able to flip the coin of the predicament to reveal essential values and a guiding vision frustrated by the present situation, it motivates movement towards self-transcending goals. This is the meaning of the InnerView motto: *what the soul wants*. It is having the capacity to see persons through the viewfinder of their well-being and deepest values, the manifesting of which leads to fulfilling a larger life purpose.

Cognitive Therapy

There are many offshoots of the cognitive therapy model, but what they all have in common is that what we think about emotional problems and conflicts is what perpetuates them. Even major issues such as depression and anxiety can be fuelled by self-talk in the form of internal convictions subliminally repeated. These self-statements reflect irrational beliefs and negative assumptions about oneself in relation to the realities of the world, and in turn become automatic self-fulfilling prophecies reinforcing the original schemas (e.g., "people don't appreciate what I do for them"). This kind of thinking is often characterized by overgeneralization, whereby the part blankets the whole. External events, such as romantic disappointments, are perceived through a filter of preset conclusions (e.g., "I am not worthy of being loved") which do not follow logically from actual experience. This irrational template leads to exaggerated painful feelings and self-sabotaging behaviours, which become funnelled into a downward spiral. With the help of reality checks from a therapist, the self-talk can be turned around. By becoming aware of counterproductive thoughts and perceptions in reaction to certain triggers, people can choose to consciously change how they interpret those events and produce different, less upsetting emotional and behavioural outcomes (Duncan, 2005).

From the InnerView perspective, the cognitive approach can ensure the head is aligned with the heart and both congruent with what the soul wants. It can also provide sound, self-reliant antidotes to destructive family, social, cultural, or religious belief systems. Yet behind every clinical case study lies a life story. Behind every life story are the histories, tragedies, comedies, and mythologies of humanity itself. Together with the client, we are on an InnerView journey whenever literal sequences are set against far-reaching horizons of evolution and the person is viewed in that context. The Latin origin of the word context, combines *con* and *texere*, meaning "to weave together". The context of InnerView Guidance refers to the process of weaving together physical, emotional, mental, and spiritual elements which form the whole person. Surface consciousness has access to only a small fraction of our holonomic capacity. The full spectrum of personhood is available when attributes of personality are to qualities of soul what waves are to the ocean.

Techniques of cognitive therapy can provide guidance for the challenge of taking a new path. Abuses of the past are recast as catalytic agents for the hero's journey. Cause-and-effect explanations of events are rewoven into a tapestry of other pathways. Deficits of character and distortions of personality are transformed into fodder for soul growth. Giving away personal power to addictions, toxic conflicts, and codependent entanglements can be salvaged by having a self-transcending purpose, in service of the whole human community. Regression and relapse are reframed as the inevitable tests and hardships encountered on an archetypal quest. Even perceived tragedies can be transformed into redemptive comedies, as Frye suggested in the *Anatomy of Criticism* (Frye & Denham, 2006).

Narrative Therapy

All therapies have their underlying premises. In narrative therapy, personal reality is shaped by the stories we tell ourselves and others. We make sense of ourselves and the world through language. Language forms the structure of meaning we ascribe to our histories and is the filter through which we understand the social sphere surrounding us and the events of our lives. Life is made of stories and stories make up life. They shape our experiences of it. We are all authoring our own living biography that circumscribes who we are and what we can be. It accounts for the past, shapes the present, and provides a blueprint for the future. Families, cultures, and nations have unique biographies as well, which in turn are situated within the overall story of humanity itself. From the perspective of narrative therapy, some stories are more conducive to an expansive and evolutionary view whereas others are self-limiting and prone to problem-saturated stasis. Narrative therapists help re-author thin or psychologically impoverished histories by eliciting the themes of heroism and resiliency that each life holds. Resource-rich alternate stories and positive arche-types displace the old tales of woe with new tales of creative, daring pathfinding (Duncan, 2005).

From the InnerView perspective, the narrative approach promotes the scope of soul growth. The ego-directed sequence shifts to self-transcending themes. Outer forces are recast by inside stories, enliv-ened by metaphors, analogies, allegories, archetypes, and myths. We are open to the full spectrum of the collective imaginative legacy, and the contextual tapestry in which the individual life of the soul is woven. The vertical dimension of life intersects with horizontal plot-driven, ground level experience and gives the literal story deeper meaning. It also gives the person an expansive identity. InnerView resembles the narrative approach when we walk the client through the rough-edged landscape of life circumstances towards its unconsidered horizons, including any transpersonal, archetypal, or spiritual realms which may be meaningful to them (Hillman, 2009). Each person is seen as the author of their own life (White & Epston, 1990). Hope is inherent in the way they can write the next chapter of their heroic story. Personal guidance leads to the inner view of a larger landscape, beyond following blow-by-blow descriptions of the plot. The singer/songwriter Bob Dylan suggested that it is an error to focus on the immediate dramas of life alone (Dylan, 1973).

We can deprogram the old histories and plotlines by reopening the story to new creative possibilities, themes, meanings, and forms of self-mastery. The error to clearly learn is the powerlessness of feeling con-fined to a psychological plot determining a fixed fate. Personal identity can be a burden and prone to dysfunction when it is reified rather than fluid and multi-faceted. This is when practitioners can experience clients as concrete thinkers, without a vision beyond the evident facts of their life situation. In narrative therapy, those facts are part of what is called a thin story. Yet subjective reality is a narrative construct. Our very sense of self belongs to a story and that story can be thickened with memories, dreams, reflections, allegories, chronicles, archetypes, and mythologies. These are all the imaginative tapestries out of which life is woven; every-thing that makes human consciousness rich, rather than impoverished and limited. The description and creative re-description of who we are, what we are, and why we are is not summarized by an aimless chronology of events. Those events are dramatic masks for the archetypal ideas, myths, personas, perspectives, and purposes that are at work in the epic story of the soul's journey. Part of our job as helping professionals is to listen deeply for those other levels and dignify the sequence of events by making what is absent in the reported plotline, present. It is where the vertical dimension of life that gives it meaning, intersects with the horizontal "this happened, then that happened . . . " ground level experience. When we serve a story in this way, it expands the client's sense of identity. Otherwise the ego remains closed to other possibilities of being, and a neurotic pattern or banal plot is "all that you've got".

In the InnerView process, practitioners serve as tour guides for new territory, as the client steps out of one story and into another, lending a future to the past that it heretofore never had. The re-telling of the story allows plotlines to form a meaningful narrative as we deconstruct the old story and co-construct a new one.

Here is an example of how an InnerView practitioner working online coached a woman who felt much trepidation after separating from her husband, because it meant setting out on her own. She was not sure she could cope. Ralph Friesen, an online counsellor and contributor to Chapter 7 in this book, offered this analogy:

> Your leaving could be compared to the flight of a refugee. When refugees leave their home, it is not because they do not love their country. They leave because their situation has become unbearable for them. If change has not been possible, and the opportunity arises, they leave. Having left, they are received in a new country. They are grateful for the kindness and support shown to them. Now, at long last, they can live in freedom. They may almost have forgotten what that is like – to be free. The very thing they yearned for so strongly is somewhat strange to them and requires many adjustments. They feel homesick for the place they have left. Yet the situation in that place is still what it was: unliveable. Emotionally, the refugee may for a time be in-between, no longer able to return to the old place and not yet able to rest easily in the new one.
>
> (Ralph Friesen, personal communication)

Positive Psychology and Solution Focused Therapy

Positive psychology, as pioneered by Martin Seligman, emphasizes personal aptitudes and capacities associated with well-being. Three domains of life to which it is applied are called the "pleasant life" (evoking positive emotions along the timeline of past, present, and future); the "engaged life" (drawing upon individual strengths and virtues); and the "meaningful life" (arising from a sense of belonging due to contributions made to the collective good) (Duckworth, Steen & Seligman, 2005).

A group of family therapists, led by Steve de Shazer and Insoo Kim Berg, preceded the positive psychology movement with a wellness-based approach they named Solution Focused Brief Therapy or SFBT (DeShazer, Dolan & Korman, 2012). De Shazer and colleagues challenged the dominant models of psychotherapy at the time, which focused on problem formation and resolution. De Shazer and his colleagues recast the role of the practitioner, traditionally positioned as an expert clinician equipped to analyse and diagnose, as more of a confidence-building coach, evoking client competencies, skills, strengths, resiliencies, successes, and resources. The approach was designed to empower clients by amplifying positive change through a focus on what is wanted (solution) versus what is not wanted (problem).

De Shazer and his colleagues referred to solution-talk as a practical method of fostering goal-setting and strength-based assessment, while reinforcing what is already working well (Iveson et al., 2012). SFBT has increasingly been hailed as a short-term alternative to what De Shazer described as "the traditional focus on problem formation and problem resolution that underlies almost all psychotherapy approaches since Freud" (DeShazer, Dolan & Korman, 2012). It challenged long-held clinical approaches based on problem-talk, as de Shazer and his team characterized pathology-based treatment modes (Lipchik & de Shazer, 1986). Solution building is a cocreated process which focuses on what clients would like to see change in their lives (best hopes), working towards gaining a clear picture of what that might look like (preferred future), then bridging back to signs of how it is already happening (present instances).

Positive psychology and the solution-oriented methodology have inaugurated a new wave in the helping professions. It is shifting the emphasis to people's strengths, capabilities, and personal resources, rather than dwelling on deficits and damage. The mental health field is now living up to its name in some sectors, rather than defaulting to mental illness treatment, in keeping with the pathology bias in psychiatric circles. This approach serves as a course corrector for the long history of marginalizing those whose mental and emotional afflictions differ more in degree than in kind from our own. Again, the approach is based on trusting what is right with persons, rather than relying on lengthy investigation of what is wrong with them. InnerView Guidance ascribes to this shift in perspective: from outside-in to inside-out, from conditions and circumstances to inner strengths and personal resources, from a narrow fixation on the problem to using a wide-angle lens, from coping with a diagnosis to how life can look through the view-finder of well-being.

When solution-focused methods are successful, they shift the client's focus from dysfunction and disability to sustainable strengths of character. They also emphasize what is of deeply held value in the person's world. The term solution is misleading, because it is about more than providing practical tools to fix life predicaments. Many clients feel that they do not just have a problem. They feel they *are* the problem. It is not only a matter of saying, "Let's take a closer look at this and see what you can do about it." To encourage the person behind the problem, we would instead say, "Let's take a closer look at who you are and who you are capable of being under the circumstances."

We can take it a little further. InnerView evokes the person ahead of the problem, that is, who they are becoming in response to it. Under the steady affirming gaze of the practitioner, clients realize they are not defined by their problem, any more than a flower is named by the weeds around it. In that sense, our approach allows the wholeness of the person to coexist with emotional wounds. It is no longer a battle between hope and hopelessness, because the person develops an expanding inner view of a much bigger landscape, which includes any spiritual or archetypal realms that may be meaningful to them. It is a matter of looking at human beings through a telescope instead of a microscope. With this kind of vision, we assess the positive core issue, while touching the pain of the negative one. Through a positive assessment of the client's own experience and wisdom, we glean what is true and good for them. When we speak of being solution-focused, it is not about a specific antidote to every emotional and psychological complaint. The standard solution-focused approach is encapsulated by the maxim: "It is better to light one candle than to curse the darkness."

Professional helpers are guides at the crossroads of where the client's life situation meets their life, needs, values, personal qualities, and soul's purpose. When we invoke the healthy purpose of the person ahead of the problem, we still show empathy for the client's predicament. Yet to gaze upon the essence of the person in this way, we need to see with the eye of the heart, hear unmet needs implied by the issue, and speak to the greater, genuinely heroic meaning of the client's life journey. That soft gaze involves looking from the inside-out in a deeply intuitive way, seeking the positive context in which the problem is situated. We then evoke the soul knowledge it takes to navigate that interior landscape.

References

DeShazer, S., Dolan, Y. M., & Korman, H. (2012). *More than miracles: The state of the art of solution-focused brief therapy*. London: Routledge.

Duckworth, A. L., Steen, T., & Seligman, M. E. P. (2005). Positive psychology in clinical practice. *Annual Review* of *Clinical Psychology*, *1*, 629–651. https://doi.org/10.1146/annurev.clinpsy.1.102803.144154

Duncan, B. L. (2005). *What's right with you: Debunking dysfunction and changing your life*. Deerfield Beach, FL: Health Communications.

Dylan, B. (1973). *Licence to kill*. Writings and Drawings (p. 469). St Albans: Panther.

Frye, N., & Denham, R. D. (2006). *Anatomy of criticism: Four essays*. Toronto, ON: University of Toronto Press.

Hillman, J. (2009). *Healing fiction*. Dallas, TX: Spring.

Lipchik, E., & de Shazer, S. (1986). The purposeful interview. *Journal of Strategic and Systemic Therapies*, *5*, 88–99. https://doi.org/10.1521/jsst.1986.5.1-2.88

Lü, D., Liu, H., Wilhelm, R., Jung, C. G., Wilhelm, S., Baynes, C. F., & Liu, H. (1962). *The secret of the golden flower: A Chinese book of life: and part of the Chinese meditation text "The book of consciousness and life"*. San Diego, CA: Harcourt, Brace and World.

O'Hanlon, W. H. (2003). *A guide to inclusive therapy: 26 methods of respectful, resistance-dissolving therapy*. New York, NY: W.W. Norton.

Palmer, P. J. (2000). *Let your life speak: Listening for the voice of vocation*. San Francisco, CA: Jossey-Bass.

Rumi, J., & Barks, C. (2004). *The essential Rumi: New expanded edition*. San Francisco, CA: Harper.

Watts, R. E. (2013). Adlerian counselling. In *The handbook of educational theories*. Charlotte, NC: Information Age Publishing.

White, M., & Epston, D. (1990). *Narrative means to therapeutic ends*. New York, NY: W. W. Norton.

2 The Presenting Person

From Treating Problems to Freeing Persons

In traditional therapy, the presenting problem takes precedence in the first meeting between client and therapist. The client is usually looking for relief from symptoms, while the therapist is looking for preliminary signs of the core issue. To serve both purposes, clients describe the details of their problematic life situation. Attention is paid to "where it hurts" in keeping with the medical model. There may be further inquiry into underlying issues such as past trauma, chronic addictions, abusive relationships, and family dysfunction (MacKinnon & Michels, 1971). While not discounting these clinical issues, a practitioner trained in the Inner-View approach would assess unmet needs related to the preferred state, values implicit in the client's story, and the overarching personal credo inferred from their goals. This method of assessment is based on evaluating strengths and resources of the inclusive self (O'Hanlon, Rowan & Rowan, 2003). InnerView practitioners investigate what is right with the person rather than what is wrong with them, as medical diagnosis might. A quote attributed to William Osler says: "Ask not what kind of disease the person has; ask what kind of person has the disease."

When we elicit a vision of the preferred state, we de-pathologize the person who is hurting or in psychological crisis, and work to narrow the gap between present circumstances and a guiding vision (Arasteh, 1965). We move from descriptions of general failures to specific positive possibilities. We shift the focus from what the client does not want, to what they do want, from what feels lost to what could be gained, and from what must be released to what can be invited into life (O'Hanlon, Rowan & Rowan, 2003). In all these ways we validate "the person behind the problem" (Yaphe & Speyer, 2010). InnerView guidance evokes the potential soul growth implicit in what otherwise are perceived as debilitating psychological conditions (Hollis, 1996).

Historical Approaches to Assessment

In the nineteenth and twentieth centuries, physicians adopted and refined the scientific method of diagnosis and treatment for addressing physical disease. As a result, the medical model, with its protocols for assessment, became the accepted standard of practice. Freud, who practised neurology first, applied that model to psychological malaise. It seems reasonable that problems need to be assessed before intervening. The more accurate the assessment, the more effective the intervention is likely to be. Psychoanalysis thus concentrated on the underlying developmental disorders and emotional complexes at the root of symptom formation. Through Freud's pervasive influence on subsequent psychotherapies, psychology in general became associated with abnormality and the understanding of mental illness. However, the linear cause-and-effect approach can be reductionistic and deterministic. It discounts that an important aspect of human nature is teleological – meaning- and purpose-driven. It overlooks that persons are motivated by intrinsic values and virtues. The medical model also keeps the expertise of the practitioner in the forefront and puts the patient in the relatively passive position of receiving treatment based on a diagnosed condition.

In the late twentieth century, psychologists Martin Seligman and Mihaly Csikszentmihalyi turned their attention above the wellness line as a corrective measure to the emphasis psychoanalysis and behaviourism placed on problematic complexes and maladaptive behaviour. Their contribution was preceded by the humanistic psychology of Abraham Maslow, Erich Fromm, and Carl Rogers, among others, which explored the roots of well-being, meaning, and emotional healing. Positive psychology was subsequently introduced in the 1980's with a focus on empirical support for what constitutes quality of life and what comprises a meaningful life. Rather than studying anxiety, depression, or personality disorders, for example, positive psychologists researched happiness, optimism, and flourishing. They examined what can go right in life and make it worth living. The professional helping relationship was re-envisioned as a collaborative endeavour, empowering clients to discover inner and outer resources within their own experience and frame of reference. The focus changed from analysing deficits to exploring assets, including strengths, possibilities, skills, values, innate virtues, and general resourcefulness within individuals and communities.

Attention then turned from theories of well-being to methods of relating to clients accordingly. This positive and hopeful approach to coaching, counselling, and therapy was named solution-focused therapy (DeShazer, Dolan & Korman, 2012). It was based in part on the observation that the more clients focused on what they wanted and valued, the more proactively they moved in that direction. The term solution in this context refers to client capacities, not specific fixes for present problems.

Most clients seeking help find themselves in painful life circumstances. InnerView guidance views their predicament as the gap between where a person is and where they want to be. Narrowing that gap involves encouraging the person behind the problem by eliciting their inherent capacities, both personally and in community. Therefore, clinical assessment includes heartfelt values, essential qualities, preferred states, underlying character traits, inner and outer resources, and any sources of hope. It is based on the confidence that needs, values, and purposes form the psychological portrait of a person. The implications of the problem end up being a small part of that picture when a client is entrained to see themselves and their life situation in this way.

When InnerView practitioners express genuine interest in the best version of a person and want to know what matters to them, it swings the balance from coping with limitations to truly encouraging their range of capability. Solution-building is a prerequisite to specific problem-solving and begins with imagining what the soul wants. The ego wants security, significance, and belonging. The soul wants wisdom, courage, and transcendence.

A study called *Values in Action, Inventory of Strengths* (Peterson, 2006) revealed that psychospiritual values fall into three broad categories the authors called: wisdom, courage, and transcendence. Spirituality in this context invokes a person's sense of relatedness to transcendent principles. Positive psychology places equal emphasis on secular and spiritual pursuits, given the core values underlying both. Another study found that spirituality and positive psychology went hand in hand (Barton & Miller, 2015). This suggests that personal spirituality may be the foundation for positive psychology traits in most people.

Given the positive assessment of personal qualities and psychospiritual traits, the solution-focused approach promotes specific, behavioural ways to make the shift from problems to possibilities (O'Hanlon & Beadle, 1999). To that end, InnerView practitioners elicit and amplify what is working for their clients. Clients are viewed as the experts on their own lives. Whereas the problem-solving approach focuses on understanding root causes to then arrive at corrective therapeutic measures, the solution-focused approach supports what the person wants instead. It highlights aspects of goals and best hopes already in effect, explores who and what matters to the client, and encourages small instances of movement towards a preferred future or hoped-for outcome. The positive framework leads to an expanded perspective of problematic situations based on client strengths, resiliencies, and resources. This serves as an antidote to the either-or dichotomies based on states of mental health or conditions of mental illness.

The difference between the problem-centred and solution-focused approaches is summarized in the following, adapted from Bill O'Hanlon's "Solution-Based Basics" (O'Hanlon, 2000).

Traditional clinical conversations tend to:

- Rely on insight and understanding as the basis for change.
- Search for deeper roots of dysfunction or pathology.
- Focus on personal history-taking as the most relevant assessment tool.
- Emphasize cathartic expression of toxic emotions.
- Attribute social conflicts to personality disorders and traits.
- Presume unconscious agendas for resisting treatment goals and methods.
- Position the practitioner as an expert on client dynamics.

The Solution-Focused approach allows:

- Collaborative exploration between partners in the healing process.
- Clients to be experts on their own experience and needs.
- Change to happen while difficulties and challenges remain.
- Strengths, competencies, capacities, and skills to be assessed.
- New possibilities for being, viewing, and doing to be brought to the situation.
- Client motivation, personal agency, and accountability to be highlighted.
- Hypothesis and characterization to be reframed as action and description.

Solution-Oriented Methods

InnerView assessment uses solution-oriented methods to make the presenting person more important than the presenting problem of standard clinical intakes. Problems become an opportunity for soul work. If we adopt a soul-growth model of healing, then we need to look at the factors which promote it. First, we elicit a vision of the ideal outcome as a shared goal for the helping relationship. Holding that vision as a reference point, we are positioned to de-pathologize the person who is in an emotional crisis. It becomes a matter of narrowing the gap between present circumstances and the guiding vision. Is there any hope for improving the situation, looking at it differently or having a different attitude towards it? What is that based on? This is the kind of assessment which humanizes and validates the person behind the problem. In this way, InnerView guidance evokes the emergent values and purposes implicit in what could otherwise be perceived as debilitating psychological conditions. We value as hidden gift what naturally could be experienced solely as emotional injury or a psychological deficit (Hollis, 1996).

This kind of positive assessment begins with eliciting the client's preferred future and imagined state of well-being. Presenting problems are put in that context to reframe life's obstacles as stepping-stones to inner-directed goals. It redirects attention from conditions and circumstances to needs and values, using various methods of solution-oriented inquiry. Again, when we speak of solution-focused we are not invoking a specific antidote to every mental and emotional complaint. The goal of all therapy is to equip clients with the inner and outer resources it may take to meet the immediate challenge or any others they might face going forward.

The Inclusive Self

To help move a client from the narrow fixation on life circumstances, we see their life situation through the viewfinder of overall well-being. We examine how they can experience some aspect of their goal now, no matter how insignificant the glimpse of their preferred state may seem. We hear unmet needs implied by their predicament and elicit the positive context of the inclusive self, which places problematic issues in a broader perspective (Figure 2.1). We explore what the client's own experience

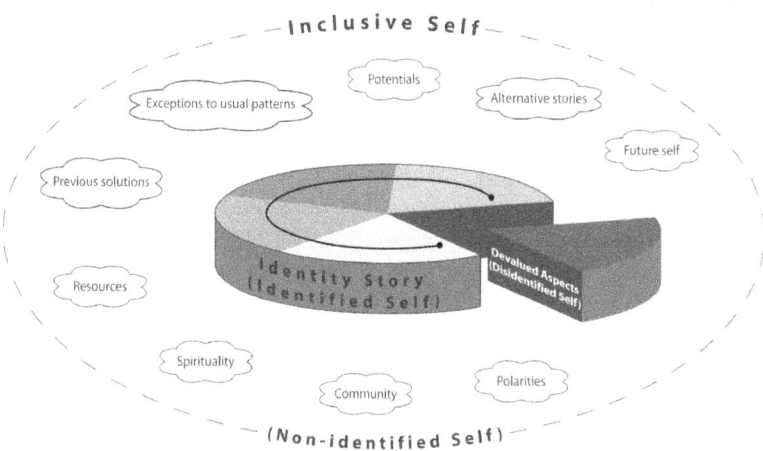

Figure 2.1 The Inclusive Self (after O'Hanlon)

and wisdom may have to say about what is true and ultimately soul-restoring for them. We want to know up front any reasons the client may have for feeling worthy of love and belonging and how they envision their rightful place in close relationships, family, and community. We look for evidence of courage (to face challenges and be imperfect), compassion (to be as kind to self as to loved ones), and connection (to become congruent with what one loves). In short, the assessment process focuses on fertile aspects of emotional, mental, and spiritual life. The field for seed-planting future changes consists of feelings, needs, values, and purposes that support soul growth no matter how much weeding of the personality may be needed.

To conduct an InnerView assessment we look for needs yet to be fulfilled, which point towards what the soul wants. We open the dialogue to values implicit in the client's story, which points towards an overarching purpose or personal credo inferred from their life goals. This approach does not discount typical history-taking, which can entail further inquiry into underlying issues such as past trauma, addictions, and self-defeating emotional entanglements (MacKinnon & Michels, 1971). However, we look at those core issues against the backdrop of the healthy big picture in which the problems are taking place. We encourage clients to separate their sense of identity from the circumstances of their unhappiness, at first by witnessing their predicament and later reinforcing a different way of being through attunement (Chapter 6).

Many clients initially present themselves as 'damaged goods'. Although the practitioner may be solution-focused, the client is likely to arrive in a problem-fixated state. Perhaps previous contact with the clinical care system has led them to say, "My depression . . ." or "I have an anxiety disorder." These are the common calling cards that clients will hand to their therapists at the beginning of their journey together. Yet when we see through the outside shell of that self-concept, we discover essential qualities at the core of client personhood (Chapter 5). In terms of the ongoing therapeutic dialogue, we are in effect sending this message: "You no more have depression than depression has you. You may experience intense emotions, think in discouraging ways, or repeat a range of behaviours that some may choose to label as a fixed condition of anxiety or depression. However, that is not you. You are Esther and this is the person I would like to get to know." It is about helping a person to feel good about themselves under circumstances that lead them to feel just the opposite.

Behind the scenes of a dysfunctional personality pattern is the potential of a person. We reframe the elements of the difficulties by looking for bright spots, or positive defiance from the problem-saturated themes. It may begin with a first impression of a client's strengths at the initial assessment. Given that many clients have been living with definitive labels such as anxiety or depression as chronic conditions, any indications of personal resiliency and positive engagement with others is a sure sign of strength. We therefore ask about who is important in their life, past or present, and the significance of those relationships. We want to hear about where their strength of character may come from and who the client thinks they resemble in their family or community in this regard. Identifying positive role models can reveal aspects of the inclusive self the client may be discounting (Figure 2.1). Where there is a problematic life situation, there are soul qualities being summoned forth to transcend or transform it. In his book *Legacy of the Heart*, Wayne Muller explores "the spiritual advantages of a painful childhood" (Muller, 2002). He reviews a series of two-choice dilemmas disrupting normal development and the courageous response it takes to achieve subsequent integration. The inner strengths summoned to overcome past suffering reveal how the original damage may have paradoxically equipped the person with psychospiritual insight and unique capacities.

Asking for Help and the Fable of the Bridge

While coping with suffering is a sign of strength, asking for help is one as well. Some clients who are seeking help for the first time may see this as a sign of weakness or failure to cope on their own. They may need to be reminded that it takes courage to recognize when help is required and to ask for it directly. It can be consoling to know that the force exerted on the lifeline by the person being lifted is equal to the force exerted by the person doing the lifting. We are equal partners although each has a different perspective from the different ends of the rope. Edwin H. Friedman's fable of the bridge presents a thought-provoking example of the helping relationship from both sides of this equation (Friedman, 1990).

Friedman tells the story of a man who sets off to meet his destiny. On the way, he becomes helplessly entangled with a man who plans to jump off a bridge. The man gives him one end of a rope and tells him to hang on or else he will fall and be lost. The helper asks the other to participate in his efforts to help him but the man at the other end of the rope struggles against his helper, impeding his efforts, while begging for help. The man must decide if he stays locked in the struggle or if he will let go, leaving the other to his fate, as he pursues his own destiny. Friedman suggests that we may play both roles in this story and that we have the strength to make the right decisions for our own lives.

Strengths, Resources, and Resilience

A positive assessment identifies successful patterns of coping and sources of resilience, especially when client stories are mostly about the consequences of trauma. Surviving trauma and all the pain it entailed can be reframed in terms of inner resources and personal heroism. At first, the story needs to be told to an empathic listener. Empathy comes before psychoeducation. However, the trauma narrative itself is not where hope lies and is not the best place to inspire change. The focus eventually needs to shift from the details of the damage done to a thorough review of the person's resilience and who they would like to become, despite the fallout from their traumatic histories. This can be accomplished by amplifying present-day coping skills, no matter how minor, all of which presuppose the ongoing emergence of a resilient person. Again, we are in effect sending this message: "It took courage to endure all that you survived. I believe you still have that courage and that it can help you create the life you want and deserve today. Together, we can look at ways for you to get in touch with your inner strengths, to use in the present situation."

The notion of the plasticity of the human brain suggests that new experiences create new neural pathways, which become stronger the more they are used (Merzenich, Van Vleet & Nahum, 2014). Fixating on negative experiences can reinforce negative patterns established by trauma. Focusing on post-trauma resilience can change how the person perceived what happened and how they perceive themselves now (e.g., as a hero). The therapeutic process can be diverted by the magnitude of the trauma story, and inadvertently maintain the reactions of the fight, flight, or freeze reactions of the limbic or reptilian brain. The more evolutionary functions of the prefrontal cortex are activated when attention turns from having survived irreparable damage to the possibilities of thriving as a stronger person (Badenoch, 2008).

Exploring a client's assets can also be a bridge to experiencing self-love. The InnerView practitioner may ask: "What do you like most about yourself and what do others like best about you?" If the client has a partner we could ask, "What first attracted your partner to you and you to your partner? What do you love most about each other now?" Naming positive qualities is an initial indicator of the ability to move beyond the presenting problem. Questions are formed to elicit what matters most to the person, thereby evoking implicit needs which in turn reveal values and purposes.

Clients are also encouraged to discuss resources available to them. For those who feel alone and unsupported in their struggle, it can be encouraging to realize that they have a support system to call upon. There may be those close at hand who would be glad to help in some capacity: a caring partner, adult children, close relatives, friends, and trusted coworkers. The client may be asked how each of these relationships normally sustains them when things are going well, and in what ways they have been there for others when needed. This kind of inquiry plants the double seed of suggestion that the client does have a network to rely upon and has made their own contributions to it. Emphasizing self-care is also part of appreciating the whole person; one not defined by the difficulties they are going through.

Assessment Includes What Is Not Said

InnerView assessment includes what the client is not saying. It is natural for anyone to be preoccupied with the problematic issue, especially in a first session. We may not hear what clients have going for them when the self-reporting is mainly about what is going against them in their life situations. In the name of active listening, practitioners risk colluding with an issue-based, blow-by-blow account of grievances. They may miss the chance to do a thorough positive assessment, which is crucial to encouraging the whole person. For example, when conducting a thorough positive assessment, we invoke qualities, skills, creative gifts, and proven loyalty clients have demonstrated to themselves over the years. We may ask about those in the client's past who believed in them and what that says about the client's present ability to overcome similar difficulties.

In containing the issue within the context of the client's best qualities, the InnerView practitioner can ask about a time when the client overcame similar circumstances or experienced some relief from it. This type of inquiry is designed to illuminate social supports as well as invoke emotional self-reliance. The potential resolution of the issue can be discussed from the perspective of the future or from a loved one's point of view. This approach can have an empowering effect, due to the genuine respect the InnerView practitioner demonstrates when assessing what is right with the person, rather than diagnosing what is wrong with them. To elicit positive self-regard, InnerView practitioners might ask clients to recall a time when they felt good about themselves and then ask, "What made it so good? How did you sense it was life-giving for you?" For future grounding as the need arises, the client can choose an image, object, or motto that reminds them of that experience and anchors it in their body or emotions. Then when they feel destabilized for any reason, they can invoke the anchor to regain emotional equanimity.

The Power to Change

Instead of staying organized around the problem, inherent personal virtues needed to transform the client's life situation can be called forth from the intrinsic wisdom and wellness to be found in full personhood. It helps to know how clients dealt with similar challenges in the past, when they managed to overcome them. We also want to find out when clients feel free from the problems in the present, if only for a moment. What makes that possible? What characteristics of the clients are involved? What do these instances of success tell the clients about themselves? What changes would they see if these successes happened more consistently? How would that fit the client's preferred mode of being? What difference would it make to their self-understanding and relationships? How does such success feel? How is that feeling experienced in the body? How can the feeling be memorized and anchored? (O'Hanlon & Beadle, 1999)

The psychological aspect of psychospiritual assessment is based on investigating anything that elicits the person's capacity to respond to circumstances with self-confidence. Therefore, practitioners delve into the personal qualities it takes to face challenging life situations.

Spiritual Resources

The spiritual aspect of psychospiritual assessment is an ongoing process of actively inquiring about a client's spiritual resources as well as their experience in religious domains. This can take the form of an implicit assessment of the sources of meaning and purpose for an individual and how they envision the sacred. Or more explicitly asking about any spiritual paths and practices, faith traditions, and religious legacies which are important to the person. These are the kind of assessments that Kenneth Pargament recommends in his book *Spiritually Integrated Psychotherapy* (Pargament, 2007). Both levels of individuation, psychological and spiritual, are enriched by images, metaphors, symbols, and archetypes. These point beyond the personal to the individual and collective stories of soul work.

When establishing connections with the person behind the problem, InnerView practitioners may identify the issue as something many of us, by virtue of being human, have experienced. To underscore that we all share the same human condition, we might muse that everyone is a slow learner when it comes to changing personal patterns, or that we are all prone to awkwardness in relationship. When we presuppose interpersonal solidarity in this way, it promotes a sense of being equally respected. We all have the same underlying need for belonging, significance, and a sense of meaning in our lives. What is unique to the individual is how he or she seeks to meets those needs. The emphasis on personal agency postulates inside-out therapeutic movement and fosters soul growth. Instead of the cause-and-effect model which can leave clients in the victim position, the InnerView model invites clients to be the cause of a desired effect by holding intentions rooted in what the soul wants. Then, as new ways of being come to fruition, the steady outgrowth of those intentions gain ground over feelings of powerlessness.

All troubles come with built-in soul tasks and personal transformation is asked of us in response to them. Psychospiritual practitioners first empathize with the felt pains of a challenging life situation; then help clients listen to what the drama of their own lives may be telling them. InnerView applies the wisdom of the ages to know how to navigate present life passages. We meet behind-the-scenes of any life drama to view what is showing up on the larger evolutionary screen. It is the humble attitude of respecting what life can teach. InnerView practitioners lead the process while deferring to the promptings of the client's own soul knowledge. There are two crucial questions involved in any soul journey. Where are we on our path? Where do we need to be? It is a privilege to accompany someone through this interior terrain as they honestly live with these questions. It is also humbling because the ultimate destiny of a soul is not ours to know.

References

Arasteh, A. R. (1965). *Final integration in the adult personality: A measure for health, social change, and leadership.* Leiden: Brill.

Badenoch, B. (2008). *Being a brain-wise therapist: A practical guide to interpersonal neurobiology.* New York, NY: W. W. Norton.

Barton, Y., & Miller, A. (2015). Spirituality and positive psychology go hand in hand: An investigation of multiple empirically derived profiles and related protective benefits. *Journal of Religion and Health, 54,* 829–843. https://doi.org/10.1007/s10943-015-0045-2

DeShazer, S., Dolan, Y. M., & Korman, H. (2012). *More than miracles: The state of the art of solution-focused brief therapy.* London: Routledge.

Friedman, E. H. (1990). *Friedman's fables.* New York, NY: Guilford Press.

Hollis, J. (1996). *Swamplands of the soul: New life in dismal places.* Toronto, ON: Inner City Books.

MacKinnon, R. A., & Michels, R. (1971). *The psychiatric interview in clinical practice.* Philadelphia, PA: Saunders.

Merzenich, M. M., Van Vleet, T. M., & Nahum, M. (2014). Brain plasticity-based therapeutics. *Frontiers in Human Neuroscience, 8,* 385. https://doi.org/10.3389/fnhum.2014.00385

Muller, W. (2002). *Legacy of the heart: The spiritual advantages of a painful childhood*. New York, NY: Simon & Schuster.

O'Hanlon, B., & Beadle, S. (1999). *A guide to possibility land: Fifty-one methods for doing brief, respectful therapy*. New York, NY: W.W. Norton.

O'Hanlon, W. H. (2000). *Solution-based basics*. Retrieved from www.billohanlon.com/LazyMan/files/solution-based-basics.pdf

O'Hanlon, W. H., Rowan, T., & Rowan, T. (2003). *Solution-oriented therapy for chronic and severe mental illness*. New York, NY: Norton.

Pargament, K. L. (2007). *Spiritually integrated psychotherapy: Understanding and addressing the sacred*. New York, NY: Guilford.

Peterson, C. (2006). *A primer in positive psychology*. Oxford: Oxford University Press.

Yaphe, J., & Speyer, C. (2010). Using email to enrich counselor training and supervision. In K. Anthony, D. M. Nagel, & S. Goss (Eds.), *The use of technology in mental health: Applications, ethics and practice*. Springfield, IL: Charles C. Thomas.

3 Living in a Bigger Story

Life Stories Re-envisioned as Soul Journeys

The InnerView vision positions the helping professional as a "guide at the crossroads" where different dimensions of life intersect. The crossroads is where the crux of life's contradictions and paradoxes is acutely felt (Williams, 1989; de Waal, 2003). The bigger story is also where the foreground and background of life's challenges are equally present. It is the perspective from which any problem takes place in the larger context of a soul's sacred story (Pargament, 2007). The person can then discern what ongoing soul formation could emerge from present challenges (Gallagher, 2012). We explore what the client's experience and wisdom have to say about what is ultimately soul-restoring for them. We want to affirm that the client is worthy of love and belonging and help them envision their rightful place in the human community. We look for evidence of courage to face challenges, practice compassion, and become congruent with what one loves.

What would characterize the awareness of a person informed by larger infinite meanings, not limited to the immediate contingencies of day-to-day existence? That person would have a bird's eye view of reality and not be mired in the worm's eye view that lacks the capacity to step back from the immediate circumstances of their lives. They would intentionally engage the heights and depths of their humanity through the wide-angle lens of consciousness. It is the difference between a divergent form of attention, at risk of becoming scattered and ineffectual, and a convergent awareness that aligns physical, emotional, mental, and spiritual levels of being.

In the physical realm, we tend to deny mortality and defend against death with self-serving strategies for happiness. The bigger story involves giving oneself to projects and causes which benefit the next generations. In the emotional realm, we tend to be absorbed in the drama of attachments, often bound up with projections of the shadow self. Yet we might also claim the freedom to navigate the complex dynamics of close relationships while anchored in unconditional love (Welwood, 2007). Mentally, in the egoic state, we are prone to thinking in either-or categories. The broader view of the soul's truth is inclusive and rooted in underlying values such as honesty, courage, kindness, and compassion. In the spiritual realm, we may identify with an idealized self. When that self-concept is split off from human limitations, it may lead to illusions of invulnerability and superiority. In the bigger story, we tap into archetypal sources of personhood that we all have in common yet express in unique ways.

Going to the Crossroads

As we grow in consciousness, each of us goes to the crossroads, willingly or not, to find our way forward. The crossroads is where the horizontal dimension of life (the interpersonal, social, and political) intersects with the vertical dimension (the transpersonal, ethical, and spiritual). It is where day-to-day decisions influence the integration of individuals, families, communities, as well as the evolution of the world at large. From this perspective, there are no insignificant gestures or moments. This is where overarching wisdom is needed to embrace life's contradictions instead of polarizing them. This approach helps expand the client's sense of identity by exploring where the linear progress of life meets the eternal dimension. When a client connects interiorly with the essential qualities of truth, beauty, and love it can help make even their seemingly intolerable experiences meaningful and potentially transformative (Hollis, 1996).

The InnerView practitioner helps persons understand they are being summoned to explore the interior landscape where the demands of a life situation take place. That is what we call soul work. We look for the soul strengths being called forth, and the essential qualities struggling to emerge in a person's unique way of grappling with circumstances. The InnerView practitioner is always asking the same question, customized to the feelings, needs, values, and purposes of the client: what capacities are needed to stay on the growing edge of this life situation? InnerView guidance is the process of eliciting those innate strengths and bringing the essential traits informing them to the fore. This is how a client's inner and outer worlds can become more congruent. It is the landscape of what the soul wants when informed by the nuanced voice of wisdom. No matter how brief or long-term, it is a therapeutic journey from present predicaments to preferred states and from conditioned patterns to empowered choices.

Freedom for Growth

There is a shift in the balance of power between ego and spirit when we achieve freedom *from* depression, anxiety, addictions, codependence, and other presenting issues. Yet there is a further step for soul growth beyond symptom relief; it is freedom *for* the contribution we can make to the world in our local sphere of influence. In the InnerView approach to healing we seek congruence between the interior landscape of what the soul wants and the life purpose we are meant to manifest in the world. The paradox is that we need to look *within* to see *beyond* ourselves. Inner transformation is reflected in outer manifestation. We look beneath the surface of life circumstances and put mental health in the context of the overarching perspective of soul work. Ira Progoff recommended a first step in this direction when he said: "As the work proceeded it became apparent that the empirical data for holistic depth psychology are to be found not in case histories but in life histories" (Progoff, 1983).

Depending on the client's spiritual orientation, the interior journey could be framed in terms of a quest for deeper meaning, the result of a personal awakening, or a desire to grow closer to that which they call God. Given client readiness from any of these perspectives, InnerView guidance connects persons with their inner voice of wisdom, maps out the terrain of their psychospiritual life, and brings more clarity to their life purpose. Along the way, clients learn to claim their strengths and self-worth and engage with others authentically. They situate where they have been, where they are, and where they are going on their psychospiritual path. They embrace their imperfect human nature and view their life situation through the viewfinder of well-being, using a wide-angle lens. They practise expanding rather than contracting their emotional capacity when facing challenging life circumstances. They explore inner and outer resources to overcome obstacles on their own path. They feel they are an integral part of an evolving human community. Through mindfulness practices, they learn to access the inner calm and confidence that helps them connect with their values.

The genuinely religious imagination (from the Latin word "religare" meaning to tie, bind together) seeks to embrace the contradictions of life, with its order and chaos, comedy and tragedy, reality and revelation. The ego's tendency is to polarize these apparent opposites. From the soul's point of view, the dichotomies are contained within a unified field. Our personal perspective takes place in a landscape of transpersonal and archetypal realms. With that shift in consciousness, we then survey the inner terrain for the soul growth we want to nurture.

Risk of Spiritual Bypassing

Spirituality without the kind of psychological integration InnerView represents is plagued by the prevalence of "spiritual bypassing" when genuine soul work is disregarded (Welwood, 2007). It is what happens when developmental processes are overlooked, often under the sway of spiritual leaders with vested interest in the immaturity of their followers (Wilson, 2000). There are various ways in which ordinary, developmental stages of maturity can be displaced by high-minded denial of shadow elements in the psyche.

John Welwood was one of the first to draw attention to developmental process skipping. "The attempt to use spiritual ideas and practices to avoid dealing with emotional unfinished business – notably our woundedness around love," he writes, "usually has disastrous consequences, especially in the West, frequently leading to psychological imbalance and destructive behaviour. My term for this kind of dissociation and denial is spiritual bypassing" (Welwood, 2007). The balanced alternative is to embrace the contradictions of life while holding a creative tension between our limits and potentials (May, 1995). Archetypal psychology has emphasized that we cannot explore the heights of life without delving honestly into its subconscious depths (Hillman, 2013). All genuine religious experience points towards becoming fully human in this way.

Containing the Dichotomies

Whether in social, political, or religious spheres, we see the fallout from dichotomous thinking in the polarized worldview of win or lose, good guys and bad guys, and us against them. Such duality has its roots in the ancient conflicts that pit faith against science, and ego against soul, for example. Lost is the integration of opposites we find whenever cooexistent qualities such as compassion and detachment are held in creative tension (Figure 4.2). When opposing ideas or clashing energies of all kinds collide within us or in society, we are naturally aggrieved. We tend to keep a tight grip on our emotional position and mentally or literally expel that which threatens us. Most of human history charts the violent power struggles that result from opposing and entrenched stances. Sacred history, both individual and collective, shows a third way of integration and synthesis, which is the antidote to the escalation of polarized grievances. It takes creative courage to maintain rather than escape the contradictions inherent in human reality. The intention of living in a bigger story is to resolve splits in the psyche. It is the way of, Buddha, Jesus, Maimonides, Jalaluddin Rumi, Mahatma Gandhi, Thérèse of Lisieux, and Etty Hillesum, among other spiritual heroes from all traditions.

Applying this dialectic to contemporary psychology brings us back to our therapeutic role as guides at the crossroads of developmental crises in the lives of our clients. It returns us to the study of redemptive values tempering the due diligence of clinical diagnosis. In practice, we apply the full scope of clinical expertise to the negative core issue. This is the glare of the assessment phase. Yet it is offset by a positive gaze on client strengths. While the glare provides valuable insight into self-defeating attitudes and problematic patterns, the gaze is focused squarely on the intrinsic capacity of persons to overcome, transform, or transcend painful life circumstances. It is a matter of remaining ever-alert to the intersection of the vertical and the horizontal dimensions of life. That is where the psychologically synergistic and synchronistic events take place. That is where we can show our clients, through the circumstances of their lives, that every problem exists as a means to call forth qualities from the gifts within. It suggests to clients that their perceived misery may have meaning, that healing may be hidden within the disease, and that every problem contains the seeds for potentialities of the soul. Larry Culliford, in *The Psychology of Spirituality*, reframed the pressure of seemingly intolerable life situations in this way: "The thrust of a rocket must reach extreme levels for it to escape the pull of the earth's gravity. Similarly, an irrepressible force is required to shift a person outwards, out of their comfort zone from within the safety of their group" (Culliford, 2011).

Promoting Well-being

There are essential qualities and a code of personal values that many clients discover on their way to an increased sense of well-being. These values have a transpersonal effect. They are the ones inspiring self-transcendence, from shamanic tribal initiations, to religious sacraments, to the moral transformations in inspirational movies. On one level, it means sorting through the inheritance of family upbringing and social conditioning for the values we want to keep. Yet it is also about living in a bigger story, which means participating in the movie scenes of life without completely identifying with one's role or getting lost in the drama. It involves the capacity to answer the call beyond oneself, which harkens back to what previous generations called character formation (Brooks, 2016). The voice of intuitive wisdom within each of us resonates with moral and spiritual guideposts from the wisdom traditions, validating our deepest sense of identity (Bourgeault & Moore, 2003). When clients rediscover qualities within themselves which align with timeless spiritual truths, it helps them live in a bigger story than the one they have been telling themselves. InnerView guidance links personal therapeutic insights to what it means to be fully human at this stage of our evolution and beyond. Sebastian Moore, a monk and mystical theologian, writes, "A total restructuring of our knowledge is required once you accept this new definition of a person: A person is a relationship of which the other is infinite" (Moore, 1981). He then asks: "What will the Psychology

Department make of that?" A Psychology Department with InnerView Guidance in its curriculum might say that the full understanding of personhood is a question of spiritual magnitude. Students would be taught that human potential outreaches the scope of what psychological theory alone can fathom.

On the personal level, we can deal with difficulties more effectively when we see troubles as a form of psychospiritual training. It is a way of living from the inside-out, by welcoming life challenges as contributing to our ultimate good when we perceive them as such. Genuine spirituality usually includes an awareness of timeless truths that reorient us in the face of adversity. Where there is a view to the good, the true, and the beautiful, there is a way to trace back the radiance that shines like refracted light through the stained glass window of personal and social conditions. It begins with attuning the client to their preferred state. Then the course of therapy becomes a matter of helping the client to narrow the gap between their current mode of being and the goals of self-actualization posited by Abraham Maslow. Colin Wilson, in his book *New Pathways in Psychology: Maslow & the Post-Freudian Revolution*, extends Maslow's ideas to consider the untapped potential of human consciousness (Wilson, 1979). InnerView practitioners encourage self-compassion for the gap between who we are and who we could be. From there, we look for inner and outer sources of renewal, ego-soul congruence, and life purpose. Given client readiness, we begin building on strengths and identify any allies in the person's own world or role models they may have in the worlds of literature, film, sports, or religion. With these essential touchstones, we are equipped to translate feelings into needs, needs into values, and values into purposes for the direction forward, no matter how tentative. The universal hope is that personal growth and collective evolution are advanced by both favourable and painful life circumstances when we see ourselves on such a journey.

The Contribution of Religious Traditions

This process has deeply meaningful reference points for those identifying with a formal religious tradition. With these clients, it behoves the InnerView practitioner to have a comprehensive understanding of the resources, pathways, and destinations within the major religious traditions (Pargament, 2007). Given this competency (Vieten & Scammell, 2015), we can then reflect upon ways in which aligning the inner self more congruently with one's contribution in the world, gains universal significance. For example, in the Jewish tradition, the individual participates in *tikkun olam*, or the repair of the world at large through specific self-giving in community. In terms of Christian faith, the central events of crucifixion and resurrection symbolize the renewed life of the soul arising out of the freely accepted diminishments and deaths of the ego. In the Islamic tradition, surrender of self-interest ushers in the dignity and worth of full moral stature. The mystical Sufis speak of a true human being who is no longer self-divided and whose human nature is consequently devoted to divine inspiration. In Hinduism and Buddhism, the person participates in the cosmic interplay, recasting a worldly sense of self. Many choosing paths outside these religious traditions, yet often featuring reconfigurations of them, prefer generic understandings. The self-concept inspiring the psychospiritual journey goes by many alternative names: spark of the divine, higher self, inner teacher, original nature. Whatever the entry point to the bigger story is called, it allows seekers to become whole, surrendered, awakened, and devoted.

The Role of Myth

The epic stories of myth and religion are often reflected in the heroic journey of healing on a personal level. We identify with larger-than-life characters, not simply because we are fascinated by their exploits, but due to the archetypal qualities they represent. Those are the same qualities we need to tap into when facing challenges which summon inner resources to the surface. Every life has its own personal mythic structure. Behind every life story are the histories, tragedies, comedies, and mythologies of humanity itself. We serve the bigger story whenever the literal sequence takes on a larger theme. This perspective serves the transition from merely coping with the immediate terrain of a life situation to a vision of self-transcending horizons. Our deeper sense of self includes mythic symbols, sacred histories, cultural inheritances, and universal archetypes; indeed, everything that makes human consciousness rich, rather than spiritually impoverished.

We know all too well what it is like to act like smaller persons in a mood of grievance repeating the same emotional patterns while expecting someone or something to rescue us from ourselves. Starting in childhood, we inevitably create stories based on the events of our lives, to make sense of our experience. Some of these stories serve us well in adulthood; others represent the damage done to us by early trauma and the personal disempowerment that often results. The voice of the painbody (Tolle, 2018) reinforces feelings of deficiency. It persuades us that there is no escape from the stuck places. Our brains are wired to tell the same story about life events which then triggers the same unhelpful coping mechanisms (Cozolino, 2002). Yet none of that defines who we are, what we are, and why we are beyond deterministic conclusions.

The Hero's Journey

From the InnerView perspective, significant life episodes are dramatic masks for archetypal ideas, guiding visions, and inspirational stories, all of which inform the soul's psychospiritual journey. Limited plotlines can be redrawn within a larger archetypal structure, reframing personal concerns in the bigger picture of what life needs from us. Then, depending on how we direct our attention, we can re-tell formative stories to include creative possibilities and emerging aspects of self-mastery. We can reclaim the shaping of our future through how we direct our attention. Our humanity is best expressed by what we do in the gap between stimulus and response, a freedom most animals do not experience, as far as we know. Yet to responsibly exercise that freedom we need to move beyond the undifferentiated, conditioned phases of psychospiritual development, to integrative and generative stages (Wilber, 1999). Each progressively developmental state represents an increase in our capacity for both vulnerability and authenticity. We always have the choice of whether to expand or contract in response to the tests of life.

The mythologist Joseph Campbell found that all myths are variations on a single story. He calls the hero's journey the monomyth (Campbell, 1949). The hero goes through three main stages, each of which has a number of sub-stages, including separation, initiation, and return. The structure of the story is universal and therefore can be invoked to encourage clients facing challenges in their own lives. The idea of overcoming archetypal forces represented, for example, by a domineering boss on the job or the fallout from a divorce, can be empowering. The hero's journey lends transpersonal meaning and dignity to what otherwise might be viewed as the clashes of self-interest during merely personal battles.

The archetypal heroic journey begins with the everyday life we all share before an initiating incident sets the person apart and summons a courageous response. There is some hesitation and self-doubt about answering the call. Then, often with the help of a mentor, the hero gains access to the resources, knowledge, and confidence it takes to cross thresholds of fear to face the challenges involved. The do-or-die world of potential transformation is then accepted, along with any ordeals presented by this new realm. There, the hero faces trials, commits to passing tests, and makes friends and foes along the way. He then undergoes an ordeal at the crossroads where he faces the greatest challenge with the physical dangers symbolizing life and death situations on a soul level. He experiences the consequences of surviving death and choosing life and continues to pursue his redemptive destiny. The hero returns to ordinary existence with something to restore the core values and hopes of his community.

The central analogy of the hero's journey is that every step on one's personal path is significant and sacrosanct, including the original crossing of the threshold, the struggle, and the return with higher consciousness. Similarly, the heroic client faces the most difficult life tasks in front of them with courage, even if at first it is a matter of 'borrowed functioning' from a mentor or role model. Eventually, the natural resistance anyone would undergo in crucial life transitions is confronted and overcome. One of the redemptive results is an acceptance of human imperfection, when the soul feels its worth and is equipped to be of service (Niequist, 2016). Ultimately, we are processes by which evolution proceeds when contributing to the needs of our community becomes at least as important as making individual progress. The authentic hero's journey speaks to the larger, overarching themes of resilience (we suffer, yet survive and eventually thrive), independence (we hear the call and take responsibility for it), courage (we overcome obstacles and make sacrifices for the greater good), compassion (we attend to the feelings and needs of our companions along the way), and faith (we hold the transformative vision).

This use of the wide-angle lens endows the sequence of (horizontal) events with (vertical) archetypal significance. In the therapeutic journey, the abuse of the past becomes a catalytic agent for soul-making, invoking the archetype of the wounded healer (Muller, 2002). Reductionist cause and effect explanation are rewoven into more layered stories with a new tapestry of choices available (the creative spirit). The risks of relapse are reframed as the inevitable tests encountered on the quest (the call to commitment). Mistakes made along the way are opportunities for self-compassion (the summons to spiritual generosity). The metaphorical dragons guarding the portal of new possibilities can be slayed or tamed (the transformation).

Clients turn from powerless ego narratives to the scope of soul growth whenever they identify with self-transcending strengths and sources of inspiration. InnerView guidance views the person through a prism refracting their unique spectrum of heritage, heredity, upbringing, and maturation. It then elicits the 'true colours' of individuated values and purposes. To focus on soul work, we invoke inspirational allies, heroic figures, and personal mentors. We also invite clients to explore the terrain of their inner lives through various mindfulness practices: contemplative reading, dream work, creative arts, journaling, and meditation to name a few. We want to learn more about their humanitarian ideals, spiritual perspectives, or religious beliefs. We explore meaningful connections with family members, friends, and community. There are many entry points to the story of the inclusive self (Figure 2.1). We also encourage the outflow of attention to whatever arouses gratitude, evokes humour, lends perspective, and leads to wisdom. InnerView Guidance summons the capacities which allow us to re-author our autobiographies with neither nature nor nurture having the last word. Adopting the attitude of "it ain't what you got, it's what you do with what you got", we are all works in psychospiritual progress.

References

Bourgeault, C., & Moore, T. (2003). *The wisdom way of knowing: Reclaiming an ancient tradition to awaken the heart*. San Francisco, CA: Jossey-Bass.

Brooks, D. (2016). *The road to character*. London: Penguin.

Campbell, J. (1949). *The hero with a thousand faces*. New York, NY: Pantheon Books.

Cozolino, L. J. (2002). *The neuroscience of psychotherapy: Building and rebuilding the human brain*. New York, NY: Norton.

Culliford, L. (2011). *The psychology of spirituality: An introduction*. London: Jessica Kingsley Publishers.

de Waal, E. (2003). *Living with contradiction: An introduction to Benedictine spirituality*. Norwich, CT: Canterbury.

Gallagher, T. M. (2012). *The discernment of spirits: An Ignatian guide for everyday living*. Johanneshov: TPB.

Hillman, J. (2013). *Archetypal psychology*. Putnam, CT: Spring Publications.

Hollis, J. (1996). *Swamplands of the soul: New life in dismal places*. Toronto, ON: Inner City Books.

May, R. (1995). *Courage to create*. Gloucester, MA: Peter Smith Publications.

Moore, S. (1981). *The fire and the rose are one*. New York, NY: Seabury Press.

Muller, W. (2002). *Legacy of the heart: The spiritual advantages of a painful childhood*. New York, NY: Simon & Schuster.

Niequist, S. (2016). *Present over perfect: Leaving behind frantic for a simpler, more soulful way of living*. Grand Rapids, MI: Zondervan.

Pargament, K. L. (2007). *Spiritually integrated psychotherapy: Understanding and addressing the sacred*. New York, NY: Guilford.

Progoff, I. (1983). *Life-study: Experiencing creative lives by the intensive journal method*. New York, NY: Dialogue House Library.

Tolle, E. (2018). *A new earth: Awakening to your life's purpose*. London: Penguin.

Vieten, C., & Scammell, S. (2015). *Spiritual and religious competencies in clinical practice: Guidelines for psychotherapists and mental health professionals*. Oakland, CA: New Harbinger Publications, Inc.

Welwood, J. (2007). *Perfect love, imperfect relationships: Healing the wound of the heart*. Boston, MA: Trumpeter.

Wilber, K. (1999). *Integral psychology*. Boston, MA: Shambhala.

Williams, H. A. (1989). *Tensions: Necessary conflicts in life and love*. London: Fount.

Wilson, C. (1979). *New pathways in psychology: Maslow and the post-Freudian revolution*. London: V. Gollancz.

Wilson, C. (2000). *Rogue messiahs: Tales of self-proclaimed saviors*. Charlottesville, VA: Hampton Roads Pub.

4   The 4Fold Path

A Psychospiritual Map for Navigating Personhood

A. Development and Purpose of the 4Fold Model

The 4Fold Path (Figure 4.1) describes an overarching sequence of therapeutic movement, intended to serve as template guiding the helping relationship. The diagram provides reference points for meeting clients at the crossroads of psychospiritual development and is a map of what constitutes the whole person. We keep the map in mind when grappling with ground-level presenting issues, since it is congruent with the four generic stages of clinical progress (Part B). As both the centrepiece of the InnerView perspective on the whole person and an orientation tool for InnerView soul work, it can be adapted to any helping practice.

The 4Fold Path map (Figure 4.1) is based on the logo of InnerView Guidance International (IGI) (www.innerviewguidance.com/4foldpath/). The map is framed by four compass points, designated by the terms spirit, soul, ego, and psyche. Each point will be presented in the first section of this chapter by describing what differentiates them from the others. In the second section, the CARE model is introduced as a basic template for the traditional fourfold phases of the helping relationship. As a meta-model for those phases, the unfolding sequence of witness-presence-essence-guidance is then described, along with subsets of that progression. The map illustrates how the four-step succession of elements unfolds, depending on the readiness of the client. The third section presents a case summary following a client's story through the 4Fold sequences on the map. First, we will introduce the basic axes of the map and the principles informing this framework.

When we speak of the "guide at the crossroads" we refer on the map to the intersection of the horizontal and vertical dimensions of life. The horizontal axis represents the earthly, day-to-day, practical contingencies of life (concrete and temporal). The vertical axis signifies transcendent principles giving life ultimate meaning and purpose (intangible and

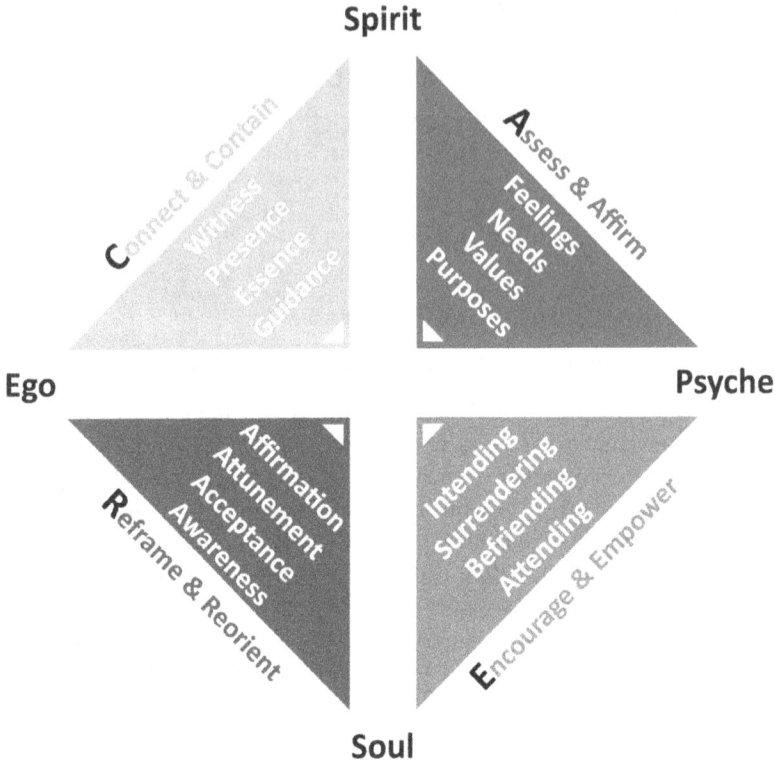

Figure 4.1 The 4Fold Path Map

eternal). The horizontal progression informs psychological work, whereas the vertical perspective is the hallmark of spiritual growth (Bourgeault & Moore, 2003). Psychospiritual development or soul work takes place at the intersection, which we call the crossroads.

That is the locus where the poles of human experience (conditioned-unconditioned, relative-absolute, psychological-spiritual, personal-universal) converge. In the words of John Welwood: "To be fully human is to forge bridges between earth and sky, form and emptiness, matter and spirit. And our humanness expresses itself in a depth and tenderness of feeling or heart that arises at the intersection of these poles" (Welwood, 2002).

To be human is to live in two worlds: the *chronos* dimension of our outer lives (horizontal axis on the map) and the *kairos* dimension of inner life (vertical axis) and to have an awareness of both worlds, or a double awareness (Stanley, 2019). We find ourselves at an in-between position in relation to all things: life and death, heaven and earth, seen and unseen. We become mature in our outlook to the extent we embrace the dialectical nature of life and its evident opposites, while seeking the synthesis of such polarities (Figure 4.2). The creative tension between the poles is universal. It is a dialectical dynamic implicit in the arts, sciences, and all forms of evolutionary endeavours. In therapy, it appears as the perceived gap between limitations and potentials, as we seek some measure of integration. The progress of our psychospiritual growth depends on maintaining double awareness and applying it to life circumstances. It becomes a way to navigate the human condition. What we call maturity is often the equanimity of a person who has learned to live with contradiction and find the third alternative between a multiplicity of dualities (Figure 4.2) F. Scott Fitzgerald reduces it to "the ability to hold two contradictory ideas in the mind at the same time, and still retain the ability to function" (Fitzgerald, 1936).

Sample Dichotomies of Life

mind ↬ body

love ↬ loss

thinking ↬ feeling

stability ↬ change

known ↬ unknown

contemplation ↬ action

fact ↬ imagination

possibilities ↬ limitations

solitude ↬ union

peace ↬ conflict

passive ↬ active

eros ↬ logos

ideal ↬ real

Figure 4.2 Sample Dichotomies of Life

The horizontal dimension involves the day-to-day, practical contingencies of everyday life. Jungian analyst Robert A. Johnson called this the "stirring the oatmeal" level of life (Johnson, 2009). It evokes the linear plotlines of a person's life journey, including all the developmental milestones along the way. The horizontal axis is comprised of the circumstances of our lives. The vertical axis represents the dimension which gives life meaning from a timeless perspective. Where the horizontal and vertical lines of movement intersect is one's present stage of psychospiritual integration. The spiritual leaders of humanity such as Moses, Buddha, Jesus, and Muhammad can be understood in this context as having reached the balanced fulcrum at the centre. Others hold it as a goal to be attained through the example and teachings of these masters.

The balancing act of being human means having a foot in both worlds (matter and spirit) while holding to the central crux of any issue at the crossroads. This is where the perspectives of spirit, soul, ego, and psyche intersect. When the archetypal components of personhood are illustrated as a map, it situates where we are internally just like longitude and latitude indicate an external location, allowing for psychospiritual assessment. By invoking a map to illustrate universal aspects of psychospiritual evolution, we have a larger context for what the soul wants. A map is not the territory. The nature of the journey is another story that the map does not presume to tell.

The four compass points on the diamond-shaped 4Fold Path graphic are spirit (north), soul (south), ego (west), and psyche (east). Mature personhood encompasses all four principles as equally as possible in a sustainable creative tension. The transcendent and numinous nature of spirit is balanced by the grounding of soul. Similarly, the more materially oriented ego is balanced by the archetypal and mythic aspects of the psyche. For the map to be useful in guiding psychospiritual growth, we need a clear understanding of what these four terms mean.

Spirit

Spirit is the fullness of life in its formless state. It is the transpersonal dimension, which many imagine as above and beyond their personal selves. From the point of view of spirit, a person is a portal through which pure consciousness takes form (as an individual soul). Anyone truly inspired has felt a connection with spirit (which comes from the Latin word for breath, *spiritus*). In many religious traditions, spirit is conceived as emanating from the heavenly realm. In humanistic philosophies and generic spiritual teachings, it is described as the animating principle within all living beings, and even things. The presence of spirit is, by definition, without definitive manifestation, because it is in the realm of the unmanifest and ultimately mysterious, given its intangible quality. In the poetic description of the Christian Bible, "The wind blows where it wishes and you hear the sound of it, but do not know where it comes from and where it is going; so is everyone who is born of the Spirit" (John 3:8). English versions of the Hebrew Bible usually translate the word *ruach* (wind) as the spirit, whose essence is divine. Similar concepts in other languages include Greek *pneuma* and the Sanskrit term *prana*. Some languages use a word for spirit closely related to mind. Examples include the German *Geist* (related to the English word ghost) or the French *esprit*. When people strive for meaning in self-transcending ways, they are being guided by the compass point of spirit.

Soul

Soul is the deepest sense of personal identity derived from a transpersonal source and as such, signifies one's unique way of belonging to life itself. It is the essential shape our personhood takes, allowing us to be *in* but not *of* the world, with its conditions and conditioning. Soul pertains to the quality of everything that grounds spirit in human experience. John O'Donohue describes the way soul is invested in all aspects of our lives in his book *Anam Cara*. He contrasts the poetics of living from the soul with the strictly clinical approach.

> In our times, the language of psychology is used to approach the soul. Psychology is a wonderful science. In many ways, it has been the explorer whose heroic adventures discovered the uncharted inner world. In our culture of sensate immediacy, much psychology has abandoned the fecundity and reverence of myth and stands under the strain of neon consciousness, powerless to retrieve or open the depth and density of the world of soul.
>
> (O'Donohue, 2004)

Spirit is embodied on the soul level, where it is grounded in lived experience. The awareness of soul purpose keeps us true to ourselves and following our destined path. Soul work enables us to resist the diversions of ego. The Christian monk, Thomas Merton, called the soul, the true self. Quakers call it the inner teacher. Buddhists call it our original nature. It is known as the Atman in Hinduism. Humanists view it as a matter of authentic identity. When we say someone has soul we are not merely speaking of character traits. It is a spiritual quality invested in the tangible goods of life, evident in the experience of soul mates, soul friends, soul food, and soul music. We feel soul connections in creative solitude, inspirational art, meaningful work, and compassionate communication. We find soul qualities wherever the surface of life meets the depths (O'Donohue, 2004).

Ego

Ego is the manager of our day-to-day experience in the world. It allows the sense of individual identity we need to function in the physical world. The ego serves us best in its executive role of making choices, setting boundaries, and achieving goals. In terms of all four compass points, it also finds its place in any life situation through the holistic work of integration. While non-dual awareness is a feature of pure spirit, the ability to differentiate the dualities of life is the province of the ego. One's whole self includes affirming the ego's worth, which is as necessary to human development as that of the body, emotions, and mind. The confusion about the rightful role of the ego is due to it being a better servant than a master. A healthy ego contributes to the fulfilment of soul purpose when it defers to the bigger stories of spirit and psyche. Otherwise, the illusion of self-sufficiency leads the ego to act as a law unto itself, unable to see beyond the narrow worldview of separateness and competitiveness. That is when the ego's preoccupation with security, esteem, and control becomes self-serving, as opposed to transformed by spiritual awareness. When the ego is in balance with the other three core components of the whole person, it empowers us to be skilful in the world. Yet this inner equilibrium depends on the ego being a servant and not a master, or as psychotherapist Thomas Moore says: "The secret of a soul-based life is to allow someone or something other than the usual self to be in charge" (Moore & Hanley, 2000).

Psyche

Psyche is the realm of the collective unconscious. It is linked to the psychologically universal. It represents the symbolic foundation of human experience, which both amplifies and depersonalizes the individual imagination (Campbell, 1949). What each of us have in common with the rest of humanity is the baseline poetics of mind. This appears in dreams, iconic images, artistic expression, and universal dramatic themes, as well as in the essential emblems of ritual, myth, and religious vision. Michael Meade, in *The Genius Myth* shows how the transpersonal power of imagination serves the interests of soul work.

> There is a poem at the heart of things and a mythic story in the heart of each of us. At certain times it is the poetry of life and the mythic

imagination of the soul that becomes necessary in order to heal the wounds inflicted by an excess of reason or an overuse of force.

(Meade, 2016)

Carl Jung placed personal imagination within the bigger story of a collective psyche. In that context dreams, art, ritual, myth, and cultural symbols reflect the universal psychospiritual motifs Jung called archetypes. He diverged from the empiricism of the medical model, thus alienating Freud, as well as from psychologies based on social adaptation. James Hillman thought Jung emphasized that the mind is in the imagination, rather than the imagination in the mind (Hillman, 2004). In that respect, psyche speaks symbolically through all things and addresses the relations of the personal and literal through the impersonal and imaginal. The richness of the psyche is our Self with a capital "S", juxtaposed to the ego self, signified by a small "s".

Clients often introduce images as shortcuts to describe their emotional pain. Practitioners employ metaphors and teaching stories to enrich the therapeutic alliance. When the wealth of teaching stories enters the dialogue, it becomes an opportunity to move from dry clinical ground to the fertile soil of psyche. The use of metaphors can make therapeutic sessions life-giving. Clients need to know they are worthy of love and respect. They need to have the courage to be imperfect and to have mercy on themselves, by learning to be self-compassionate instead of self-condemning. They need to feel connected to an outside world which is the better for their presence in it. If this could be taught didactically, simply in those terms, self-help material would suffice. Yet clients imagine significant shifts long before actualizing them. What the soul wants is often latent until increased consciousness calls it forth and brings it into view on the inner horizon. Ira Progoff described that kind of personal evolution from the viewpoint of holistic depth psychology.

> Re-entering the transitions of a life and moving from cycle to cycle within it builds a sensitivity to the inner rhythms of change. It enlarges our interior perspective of human experience and gives a larger understanding of how creative integrations take shape, often as though spontaneously, beneath the surface of events. Translated into each individual's circumstances, this understanding leads to a more developed capacity of judgment and timing, a capacity of wisdom in the conduct of life by the light of our personal values.
>
> (Progoff, 1983)

We can see what Progoff means by considering this direct feedback from a client summing it up for themselves: "I was very moved by the unique stories and analogies offered on a consistent basis to expand my understanding of the issue and show me how it looked from a broader perspective."

Given this overall orientation to the compass points on the 4Fold Path map, we can now consider the implications of psychospiritual imbalances. The direction of disintegration, dysfunction, and even pathology might be seen in the degree to which there is overinvestment in one of the poles at the expense of the other three. To use extreme examples for the purpose of illustration, someone at the Spirit pole to the exclusion of the other three, could be dissociated from worldly responsibilities and vulnerable to the seductions of a cult. Being extremely unbalanced at the Soul pole could leave someone completely identified with the extended ego of in-group ideology. It might manifest as an ethnocentric tribal mentality. A healthy, balanced sense of soul is often embodied in community, but in its overidentified, dissociated form, can lead to thinking one's culture or religion is the only one that matters, with the others posing a threat. At the extreme of the Ego pole, the person could be completely preoccupied with narcissistic strategies for seeking happiness. This usually entails valuing security, esteem, control, and power in self-serving ways. Alfred Adler, the founder of Individual Psychology, thought making a useful contribution, which he called social interest, was the key to mental health. (Adler, Ansbacher, & Ansbacher, 2006). At the extreme of the Psyche pole, losing touch with ego functioning could mean being flooded with images arising from the substratum of the collective unconscious, and placing one at risk of psychosis. Ego and psyche need the value of each other the way that spirit and soul do. The challenge is to equally embrace all elements of the human condition represented by the four compass points and their dynamic intersection at the crossroads. InnerView guidance supports that work of integration by fostering full development of all four aspects of the whole person.

B. Therapeutic Applications of the 4Fold Model

Training for most practitioners doing therapeutic work includes an overview of the process, often divided into four generic phases. In the Adlerian approach these steps are defined as engagement (establishing rapport, and empathic connection), assessment (history-taking in order to evaluate underlying core issues), insight (interpreting the roots of present problematic issues), and reorientation (guidance towards achieving developmental goals) (Watts, 2013). The analogous sequence for InnerView guidance is based on the CARE model (Figure 4.3). The phases of this model are positioned on the outer edges of the 4Fold Path map (Figure 4.1).

The CARE Model

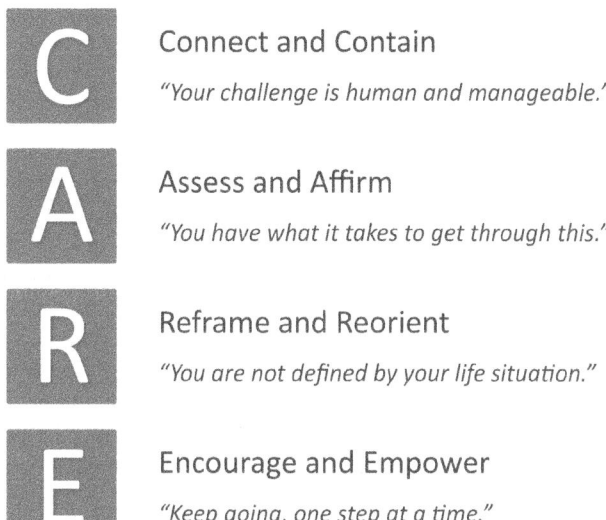

C Connect and Contain
"Your challenge is human and manageable."

A Assess and Affirm
"You have what it takes to get through this."

R Reframe and Reorient
"You are not defined by your life situation."

E Encourage and Empower
"Keep going, one step at a time."

Figure 4.3 The CARE Model

CARE stands for connect and contain ("Your challenge is human and manageable"), assess and affirm ("You have what it takes to get through this"), reframe and reorient ("You are not defined by your life situation"), encourage and empower ("Keep going, one step at a time") (Yaphe & Speyer, 2011). It is a background template for practitioners establishing rapport with those seeking support. Each phase of the CARE process can serve as a stand-alone therapeutic intervention or be a transition on the continuum of personal growth. It is congruent with any psychological theory and can be applied to any clinical approach. The steps are guideposts for the journey and not about what happens on a specific path. For example, in the body-centred psychotherapy of Christine Caldwell, the sequence for moving through addiction is awareness, owning, acceptance, and action (Caldwell, 1996). From a Jungian depth psychology perspective, the generic progression is conceived as catharsis, elucidation, education, and transformation (Jung, 1982). From the InnerView Guidance viewpoint, the sequences of the CARE model are generic and apply to the fundamentals of relationship-building, no matter what other process is taking place.

The purpose of providing an overview of the process is for the practitioner, who is leading the relationship, to have a sense of intention and direction. Part of the practitioner's job is not to get lost in the client's story and become mired in descriptions of client malaise. Remaining aware of what ideally takes place by following this sequence enables practitioners to stay conscious of their role in therapy.

Connect and Contain

The feeling of being heard and validated is paramount during this phase. Full attention is given to the client's pressing concerns. The intention is to offer empathic understanding of the presenting issues and faith in the client's capacity to resolve them. This is when the therapeutic alliance is established, based on the quality of rapport building. At this stage, the practitioner conveys unconditional positive regard for the person behind the problem and recognizes client resiliency under the circumstances. It is also an opportunity to help the client witness the predicament from a healthier emotional distance. To contain the issue within the context of client goals, we can ask about a time when they overcame similar circumstances or did not feel the issue as acutely. We can invite the client to perceive the issue from a loved one's point of view or imagine how it will look five years into the future. We can also position the issue as fading in the light of the client's true values. These interventions can have an encouraging effect, as the guide shows genuine interest in what is right with the person.

Assess and Affirm

InnerView assessment pays attention to symptoms, yet from the perspective of the soul, symptoms are viewed as harbingers of potential growth. Even if it appears to be a psychiatric disorder, from the InnerView point of view it does not have the last word on the true nature of the person. While maintaining the initial empathic alliance, the client is put in charge of underlying family rules, personal patterns, irrational convictions, or emotional habits which may have contributed to the present predicament. The assessment implies new responsibility, linked with a vision of healing possibilities. The client has choices.

Standard clinical assessment is prone to identifying the person with the problem. For example, we say a client named Julia *is* depressed. If she has received a medical diagnosis, Julia may say "I *am* depressed". Language is important. It shapes perception. Julia is still all that makes her Julia first and foremost, even though she reports experiencing depressive thoughts and feelings. The client has the problem. The problem does not have the client. The problem may not even be a problem, from another vantage point. In the end, the client is not a victim of circumstances. There can be hidden ease on the flip side of dis-ease. InnerView affirmation is a fundamental vote of confidence that the client's internal and external resources are sufficient to rewrite the story and not let negative conclusions prevail. The client is understood and appreciated for previously undervalued aspects of their development. While being careful not to minimize the pain of the issue, the guide can elicit a different story in which there is the chance to be cast in a different role. It is a remotivational approach based on an assessment of strengths. This phase is about planting the seeds of possibilities for change wherever pathologies may predominate, or a mental health condition is labelled as chronic.

Reframe and Reorient

When there is enough emotional readiness to allow for it, the practitioner assists the client in viewing the issue differently. The emphasis is on cultivating capabilities rather than eliminating difficulties. It is a time for challenging emotional convictions that do not support a vision of the preferred state. Sometimes the client resists re-evaluations of perceived negatives and the practitioner is working harder than the client. Then a variety of methods may be used. Defences can be reframed as useful coping mechanisms for the time being, pending future progress. In other words, the client can be advised to postpone change and instead accept symptoms as protective devices. Or invited to pay attention to symptoms as indicators of unmet needs (Rosenberg, 2015). The following are examples of some methods used to support shifts in perception or attitude: positive tracking of functional coping patterns, invoking hope and humour as an antidote to negativity bias, recasting perceived failures as part of the hero's journey through a series of defeats, working with metaphors, analogies, and teaching stories to reinforce the preferred state, and drawing upon sources of inspiration and meaning.

Encourage and Empower

In the concluding phase of the helping relationship, client progress is summarized and reinforced. The client's efforts towards issue resolution are validated, bolstering their potential for self-mastery. Therapeutic interventions move toward reinforcing new perspectives. If the initial phases of the process succeeded in putting the client in the driver's seat, subsequent sessions validate positive transitions in perception and behaviour the client may be making. Any paradigm shift in the client's point of view will take time to integrate. The practitioner attunes the client to the faith that he or she has what it takes and provides orientation for change. As part of reinforcing personal gains, the practitioner invokes client capabilities, by reminding them of the storehouse of strengths and resources they can draw upon going forward. There will be future challenges, however the client has what it takes to overcome them. Personal growth involves withstanding growing pains. In addressing outstanding issues, the practitioner emphasizes the corrective emotional experience set in motion. When indicated, the client is referred to some form of follow-up. Throughout the process, the practitioner aligns with the client's positive intentionality, encourages the capacity to embrace difficulties, and focuses on small positive steps. Closure is based on the client having become their own best guide and internalized the practitioner's point of view. "My voice will go with you" (Erickson & Rosen, 1991). The client is encouraged to trust her own experience and wisdom. She is the artist of her own life and the author of her own story. Significance, belonging, and meaning which we often seek outside ourselves, can be accessed from the inside. This is a central principle of InnerView.

Unfolding the 4Fold Path Map

The 4Fold Path model can be applied to any issue, though none of the elements on the map are necessarily overtly discussed with the client. It is meant to serve as a background template for the practitioner's benefit, like any map that shows how to get from where you are to where you are going. Much like learning to drive, the separate skills involved eventually become seamlessly unified. The elements appear on the map as distinct features, but in session they are all part of one process happening concurrently. For example (looking at the bottom two quadrants), given practitioner qualities of awareness, acceptance, attunement, and affirmation, the client will be learning attending, befriending, surrendering, and intending, as part of a more conscious response to their life circumstances.

All four triangles point like arrows towards the central point of integration at the crossroads. The terms within the triangles unfold in alignment with the ones on other levels sharing each triangle's position on the map. For example (looking only at the top two quadrants), when the practitioner is modelling a mindful *witness* state, it opens the space for the client to express *feelings* without fearing judgement. Similarly, the practitioner's attentive *presence* allows for the acceptance of client *needs*, whether met or unmet. In turn, a sense of the client's *essence* can elicit the *values* supporting it. Then *guidance* serves the client's *purposes*, with the latter having unfolded through a natural progression of feelings leading to needs that reveal values.

The therapeutic alliance is deepened and strengthened with each unfolding sequence of the 4Fold Path. Ideally, the more conscious the practitioner is of the meta-process and the unfolding sequences, the more the psychospiritual capacities involved will be part of the client's experience as well. Following this basic framework for a helping relationship, we can now delve more deeply into the elements named within the series of triangles pictured in the 4Fold Path map (Figure 4.1). Four double sets of four enfolding elements are posited, with the matching terms forming more of a hologram (each aspect containing the whole) than sequential steps. The first set represents states of therapeutic consciousness (witness, presence, essence, guidance) which elicit corresponding levels of client self-awareness (feelings, needs, values, purposes). The second set of parallel processes features therapeutic qualities (awareness, acceptance, attunement, affirmation) which engender successive states of client mindfulness (attending, befriending, surrendering, intending). Lastly (though not pictured on the printed map), introducing psychospiritual practices (mindfulness, meditation, creativity, spirituality) can serve to attune the client to the corresponding benefits of those practices (stillness, silence, simplicity, service). An expanded version of the 4Fold Path graphic containing that third double set of elements appears on the InnerView Guidance International (IGI) website (Speyer, 2020).

Witness (Feelings), Awareness, Attending are the spacious, nonattached states of consciousness we can bring to life dramas. It is the difference between the worm's view and the bird's-eye view. Witnessing involves the capacity to step back and take a dispassionate, observer's view of circumstances. It is like having the background awareness that one is watching a movie while still emotionally involved it. Witnessing can be entrained through meditative practices, by allowing mental and emotional activity to arise and dissipate as it will. It instils the equanimity of seeing the big picture encompassing all of life's contradictions (see Figure 4.2). It also allows for a clearer sense of the person behind the problem. Witnessing is an essential aspect of mindfulness teaching (Germer & Siegel, 2014). It fosters emotional regulation. We can feel what we are feeling without the compulsion to act on it. Activating the witness function changes how one responds to adversity because mindful attention is not solely fixated on the obstacles on one's path. It abides in a wider, deeper consciousness.

Presence (Needs), Acceptance, Befriending dissolve the duality between self and other when we hold the space for our common humanity, no matter how divergent the personalities are on the surface. With power differentials diminished by simple shared presence, healing can emerge on its own terms. In this phase, we relate to the person behind the problem, the person whose identity is not defined by life difficulties. When the practitioner brings the gift of presence to a session, it can attune the client to their true nature. The authentic expression of feelings flourishes in response to heartfelt interest in the person and empathy for the whole spectrum of their subjective experience. Presence allows the true self breathing room, which then naturally expands beyond identifying with social roles in life to the quality of life we bring to those roles. It also encourages the client to befriend negative feelings as indicators of unmet needs (Rosenberg, 2015). This approach entrains the client to allow any emotional toxicity to circulate like a parent letting overactive children run around until they tire themselves out. Soulful presence is the antidote to feeling like a victim of oneself, others, or a life situation. It is the capacity to view ourselves with the compassion we would extend towards a loved one under the same circumstances.

Essence (Values), Attunement, Surrendering allow a backstage pass to the worth of a person in and of themselves, aside from any ego strategies used to achieve belonging and significance. The word soul is shorthand for the essence of a person as opposed to the ego identity. An InnerView practitioner ideally has an intuitive sense of a person's essence or true self, described in Chapter 5 as the innermost Russian doll. In this phase, we explore any life-giving experiences or intentions that are congruent with "what the soul wants". Essence is based on the felt sense of who someone would be without mind, memory, or association. Attunement to essence is what happens when someone sees themselves with the same kind of unconditional gaze a loving mother brings to a newborn child. Feeling the undercurrent of essence allows one's heart to open and expand instead of contracting in the face of emotional pain. It allows for the self-trust it takes to go against the grain of fight, flight, or freeze reactions. InnerView attunement gives us the courage to stay present to what feels hurtful, knowing our essence cannot be damaged. Then we can afford to trace back what fear, grief, even despair have to say about how far we have strayed from our true self.

Guidance (Purposes), Affirmation, Intending apply to the crossroads where a particular life situation (horizontal axis) meets the challenge it presents for soul growth (vertical axis) and becomes a choice point. Whenever suffering can be perceived as happening *for* a person, rather than *to* a person, guidance may emerge. Guidance takes place when the perennial question of "Why me?" shifts to the inquiry, "How might I use this situation as an opportunity to find a new level of being?" By seeking to be transformed by a personal predicament rather than just suffer from it, we can make important choices more intentionally and less emotionally. Guidance then allows us to change our habitual ways of experiencing any life situation (O'Hanlon, 2015). When we ask the shadow emotions what the soul wants, intense emotional states can be translated into psychospiritual insights. Anger speaks to what needs to be protected. Guilt and shame point to what must be restored. Resentment hides the shadow side of a person until it is reintegrated. Apathy and boredom belie what matters most. Fear highlights what needs attention. Chronic anxiety and worry call for grounding skills. Confusion summons renewed intentionality. Sadness addresses the need for release and depression seeks deeper sources of creative energy. The emotions contain subtle calls to action for the consciously evolving soul since the world lives in us as much as we live in the world.

As InnerView practitioners we are privileged to serve as stewards of soul work and facilitate the fourfold sequences described previously. With the help of the 4Fold Path map, we maintain a meta-awareness of witness-presence-essence-guidance throughout the therapeutic journey. However, we also realize the map merely provides guideposts to keep us on the path. It is not meant to be a teaching tool for the didactic psychoeducation of clients. In other words, the compass points and sequence of elements are not necessarily discussed in sessions. The map is mainly intended to be a professional development tool, providing a model of full personhood for the orientation of InnerView practitioners. When clients come to us struggling with some aspect of human nature, and in some respect not feeling fully human, it helps to have an understanding and vision of what comprises the whole person. Then we meet clients at the crux of their predicament with a view to what will bring them into alignment with the core elements of their human nature.

We say an InnerView practitioner is a guide at the crossroads. A guide is not the same as a travelling companion, so every InnerView guidance relationship, no matter how short or long-term, involves handing the compass over to the client to find a direction (inner and outer) that is right for them. Our responsibility as InnerView practitioners is to encourage therapeutic movement in the direction of soul growth. We invite clients whose preoccupations collapse upon the self in involutional, unhealthy ways, to direct their attention to what the soul wants on its evolutionary journey, which is bound to be of service to others. The basic premise of InnerView Guidance, framed in terms of the 4Fold Path, is that every person has the soul work of aligning their inner and outer worlds. We trust that takes place with or without InnerView interventions. Our role as InnerView practitioners is to navigate the landscape of soul growth through unfolding sequences of psychospiritual awareness. Our goal is to support and honour what the soul wants in any relationship, especially in the helping one.

C. Case Summary: The InnerView Vision of Johanna
John Yaphe

This case study demonstrates how the CARE model and other elements of the 4Fold Path are put into practice. The CARE model is a template for the practitioner; the process translates to client experience as the sequential unfolding of *feelings*, *needs*, and *values*, leading to a deeper sense of life *purpose*. From the practitioner's perspective, Johanna's story shows how we *witness* the presenting issue in a mindful way, bring an empathic *presence* to the person behind the problem, elicit their *essence*, and evoke *guidance* associated with how the individual's story takes place in a meaningful context. These aspects of the process are presented as sequential for the benefit of practitioner training. We are always facing a whole person whose growth is organic and not subject to a series of definite steps. In the short-term context, the spontaneous emergence of the person's optimal state takes precedence over any therapeutic agenda for their progress. Names and some clinical details in this story have been modified to preserve anonymity.

Phase 1 – Connect and Contain

Johanna was a 42-year-old woman and mother of two children who was recently widowed. She worked as a human resources manager in the transportation industry. She was referred to me because of emotional difficulties interfering with responsibilities at work and at home.

Her husband had died a year ago from cancer. She thought she had managed to cope with this significant loss but recently felt "alone and disjointed with life". She was unable to focus on her work and had lost her desire to participate in activities she once enjoyed. Johanna felt she was "just trying to keep my head above water". She wanted to talk to someone but felt that no one could really understand what she was going through. She felt life was pushing her to keep moving but that she was "still stuck back there".

I was moved by the vulnerability of her situation and the emotional honesty with which she shared the aftermath of her grief. Holding the heartfelt awareness of her predicament without any judgment or even much commentary gave Johanna permission to attend to her feelings in the same way. The first step of the CARE model is to connect and contain. This facilitates the recognition and acceptance of feelings. The underlying message to the client is, "Your challenge is human and manageable." I expressed empathy for Johanna's emotional state and the challenges of day-to-day coping, especially with the care of two young boys, leaving little time for herself. I also understood her emotional turbulence within the normal context of grief and mourning. Her pain was part of the human experience of loss we all share. As I modelled unconditional acceptance, Johanna visibly relaxed into the bodily sensations of her grief, without as much of the worried story attached to it. As she befriended her feelings in this way, there was the release and relief of tears.

Phase 2 – Assess and Affirm

In subsequent sessions, I continued to support Johanna through being present to her as a whole person with all the strengths and resources she had going for her. The second step in the CARE process is assessment and affirmation. I validated Johanna as a person who could allow grief to flow through her without being trapped in it. As her trust in the process deepened, I asked more about her marriage and the values it allowed her to live out. Johanna told the story of her husband and how much she and her young sons gained from his devotion. Although she realized he was not perfect, she described her husband as "an amazing family man" whose absence had "left a hole in our lives". She told me about the palliative care he received and how he was able to die at home. She allowed herself to cry in our sessions, and share the turmoil of her mixed feelings, but felt she could not do this at home as she believed it would be a burden for her children.

I also learned more about the bond with her husband. The unspoken subtext was how this relationship was still with her, and more so because of the loss of the actual person involved. The message implied by situating the love they shared as hers to hold onto and carry forward was "You've got what it takes to get through this."

On a psychoeducational basis, Johanna was informed about the familiar stages of coping with loss, including anniversary reactions. She was reassured there was no firm timetable and that we all take this journey at our own pace. As a driven career woman with high expectations of herself, it helped to realize she had a deep need to surrender to the waves of grief she had been blocking. If she knew she was not going to drown, she could consent to landing on an unknown shore. Keeping her head above water took on a new, less threatening meaning. In terms of her worries about functioning, she understood that she could scale back her expectations of rapid progress. As a parent, she shared what a big adjustment it was to be a single mother. Naming this brought up the need for self-compassion.

Phase 3 – Reframe and Reorient

During the middle stages of therapy, Johanna travelled to another city for a professional development course. She found it hard to be away from work because she had "so many things going on". She felt her colleagues had no idea how she was feeling since she had never asked for their support. This was the first time in over a year that she had been alone, away from her family. Having space and time for herself provided an opportunity to reflect on the past year.

Johanna realized she had been hiding away from life. She had hoped taking a course with new people and hearing fresh ideas would "spark a new chapter in her life". She hated feeling lonely and recognized her need for physical and emotional intimacy. This need had led her to engage in "destructive behaviours" which included excessive use of alcohol, leading to a casual intimate encounter. She told me what she was really seeking was "a hand to hold and a hug" which she understood to be the essential need, in keeping with her moral values.

I accompanied Johanna at this stage in her journey with the third step of the CARE model in mind, which is to reframe and reorient. The implied message is "You are not defined by your life situation". It allows the client to tune into what matters to her. Since Johanna had unexpectedly become the sole caretaker of her sons, and naturally put them first, she did not feel her own needs could be legitimately met. The anger about her predicament, previously disavowed as a selfish reaction, could now be expressed and accepted as part of the grieving process. It was not something to be judged. Johanna also shared feeling ashamed of her initial attempts to "move on", perhaps prematurely, to meet her need for intimacy. Considering the essence of this need, more than the strategies she used to meet it, became another opportunity for self-compassion. Furthermore, by not judging herself so harshly in this instance, self-forgiveness became an overall theme. Johanna was learning to let herself be.

This befriending of herself could be applied in all areas of her life. For example, the very act of crying openly in our sessions was accepted and even welcomed. Perhaps her sons had the same need. She could cry at home too, to show her sons this was natural under the circumstances. She was finding it hard to tolerate their anger, but when it was reframed as another expression of grief, she saw the wisdom in allowing them to express their emotions freely. She could model the emotional atmosphere that would allow them to turn to her for support when they needed it (much like the safe therapy space had done for her). This became a breakthrough point for Johanna. When she gave herself permission to talk about her husband with her children, they discussed how they would honour his memory together.

This reorientation to her emotional life was a revelation for Johanna that led to a therapeutic step forward. So too was her openness in expressing the need for physical intimacy. It became a sign that she was ready to start reclaiming lost parts of herself. By separating the need from how she tried to meet it, she was free to choose another path more consistent with her values. In the end, Johanna felt that the time away from home on her course had helped her to see things differently. She now felt less afraid and less driven to escape her pain. It was as though a weight had been lifted.

Phase 4 – Encourage and Empower

After the turning point in our short-term work, Johanna increasingly reported the effects of her new outlook both at home and at work. At work, she had begun to confide in trusted colleagues about what she had been going through and was surprised at how much they genuinely cared about her. During this phase, Johanna came to a new sense of self-acceptance, which she experienced as a secure baseline. Upsetting thoughts and emotions no longer had to be suppressed in the name of coping, because she knew she could "ride out the ups and downs". She even found herself saying aloud, "I like me and I like my life". Knowing she would continue to heal over time, she could turn her attention to ensuring a full and meaningful life for herself and her children, as her husband would want.

Johanna raised the issue of closure with me herself, as if to demonstrate that she could handle another loss. "You are still here with me, but you won't be for long". She had begun to anticipate a replay of her grief in a manageable way, knowing she would feel "on her own" again when our sessions concluded. This new kind of loss needed processing before Johanna could move on. I participated in it by transparently sharing how I was moved by her courage and resiliency.

As if considering whether to extend our sessions, Johanna reported that she had "complicated things by meeting someone who has in a very short time become very important to me". She felt ready to have someone new in her life yet was going to be cautious and not rush into it. Despite natural fears and concerns about starting a new relationship, Johanna affirmed that "I don't need someone. I want someone."

Given the clear intention she expressed, I supported Johanna's discernment that she was well-equipped to follow through with the new relationship and had the fortitude to deal with any challenges she would face along the way. This approach is characteristic of the fourth step in the CARE model – to encourage and empower. The message to the client at closure is: "keep going, one step at a time". Johanna was encouraged to stay on the path of trusting herself, knowing she had the emotional resiliency to seek connection safely. Life still held much promise she could embrace. She was empowered to "pay forward" the steadfast love of her husband as she opened her heart to a new partner. She was reminded that she was moving forward even when it did not feel like progress. She was validated in her need to find intimacy and partnership, in a way that was a true expression of herself and not an escape. In short, Johanna had been to the crossroads and rather than it being an impasse, discovered it was the locus of soul growth.

References

Adler, A., Ansbacher, H. L., & Ansbacher, R. R. (2006). *The individual psychology of Alfred Adler: A systematic presentation in selections from his writings.* New York, NY: HarperPerennial.

Caldwell, C. (1996). *Getting our bodies back: Recovery, healing, and transformation through body-centered psychotherapy.* Boston, MA: Shambhala.

Campbell, J. (1949). *The hero with a thousand faces.* New York, NY: Pantheon Books.

Erickson, M. H., & Rosen, S. (1991). *My voice will go with you: The teaching tales of Milton H. Erickson, M.D.* New York, NY: Norton & Company.

Fitzgerald, F. S. (1936). *The crack-up: A desolately frank document from one for whom the salt of life has lost its savor* (p. 41). Chicago, IL: Esquire Inc.

Germer, C. K., & Siegel, R. D. (2014). *Wisdom and compassion in psychotherapy: Deepening mindfulness in clinical practice.* New York, NY: Guildford.

Hillman, J. (2004). *Archetypal psychology.* Putnam, CT: Spring Publications.

Johnson, R. A. (2009). *We, understanding the psychology of romantic love.* San Francisco, CA: HarperOne.

Jung, C. (1982). *Collected works of C.G. Jung, Volume 16: Practice of psychotherapy* (G. Adler & R. Hull, Eds., pp. 53–75). Princeton, NJ: Princeton University Press. https://doi.org/10.2307/j.ctt5hhr69.

Meade, M. (2016). *The genius myth.* Seattle, WA; Greenfire.

Moore, T., & Hanley, J. (2000). *Original self: Living with paradox and originality.* New York, NY: Harper Collins.

O'Donohue, J. (2004). *Anam čara: A book of Celtic wisdom.* New York, NY: Harper Perennial.

O'Hanlon, B. (2015). *Solution-oriented spirituality: Connection, wholeness, and possibility for therapist and client.* New York, NY: W.W. Norton and Company.

Progoff, I. (1983). *Life-study: Experiencing creative lives by the intensive journal method.* New York, NY: Dialogue House Library.

Rosenberg, M. B. (2015). *Nonviolent communication: A language of life.* Encinitas, CA: Puddle Dancer Press.

Speyer, C. (2020). *The 4Fold path*. Retrieved from www.innerviewguidance.com/4foldpath/

Stanley, C. (2019). *Evolutionary leap: Colin Wilson on psychology*. London: Routledge.

Watts, R. E. (2013). Adlerian counselling. In *The handbook of educational theories*. Charlotte, NC: Information Age Publishing.

Welwood, J. (2002). *Toward a psychology of awakening: Buddhism, psychotherapy, and the path of personal and spiritual transformation*. Boston, MA: Shambhala.

Yaphe, J., & Speyer, C. (2011). Text-based online counseling: Email. In R. Kraus (Ed.), *Online counseling* (2nd ed.). Cambridge, MA: Elsevier Academic Press.

5 The Matryoshka Method

An Inside-Out Approach to Clinical Process

Mental health professionals are increasingly making the transition from the traditional medical model with its focus on treating disease, to working above the wellness line using a health-based perspective. For example, during assessment, the priority is to find out what is right with the person at their core. We call this the Matryoshka Method, referring to the popular image of nesting Russian dolls. The traditional clinical assessment process seeks to gain insight into unhealthy patterns of thought and behaviour which are rooted in primary emotional wounds (MacKinnon & Michels, 1971). This approach is inherited from the medical model of diagnosing the disease in order to introduce the cure and restore homeostasis. However, when applied to therapy, treating the issue in this way can paradoxically entrain the patient to remain in a problem-saturated state of mind. The InnerView approach reverses this tendency by making the healthy nature of the person the starting point, rather than the end point (O'Hanlon, Rowan, & Rowan, 2003).

The Matryoshka Method shows how this is achieved by realigning outer personas with the essential needs, values, and intentions of the soul – the core Russian doll. Understanding the layers that are added over time through successive life experiences can also help to build a vision of strength undergirding healing and further growth. This is contrasted with the classic method of stripping away layers to look for a deeply wounded core. InnerView guidance draws upon the client's preferred state and puts presenting problems in a proactive context to reframe life's obstacles. It redirects attention from conditions to needs and values, using various methods of solution-oriented inquiry (DeShazer, Dolan, & Korman, 2012).

Soul as Innermost Essence

Soul as represented by the innermost Russian doll is the unconditioned, essential aspect of a person. It is the central worth and original blessing of personhood which cannot be reduced to biological predispositions, psychological mechanisms, or sociological constructs. The core of goodness which dwells in each of us goes by many names: true self, higher self, essential identity, deepest nature. Thomas Merton called it the incorruptible *point vierge* (Merton, 2014). Quakers call it the inner teacher. Buddhists describe it as our original nature or big self, though Zen Buddhists experience it as nameless. Judaism posits the quality of soul in every choice made between *yetzer ha-tov* (the inclination toward goodness) and the *yetzer ha-ra* (the inclination toward evil). Non-fundamentalist Christians see soul as the divine aspect of self that emerges to the degree one emulates and participates in the spiritual surrender of Jesus. Many individuals are out of touch with this inner core of goodness and depend on appearances for self-worth. There are countless examples of those whose public image has been successfully constructed, yet who remain personally dissociated and interpersonally disconnected.

Many can relate to the experience of feeling like a different person in the presence of different people. A coach or mentor can bring out the best in me while in the presence of another person I find I am not at all myself. People tend to live up to as well as live down to others' perceptions of them. This has implications for human relations of all kinds. Children tend to fulfil adult expectations of them for better or for worse, with other factors such as intelligence and aptitude being equal (Benner & Mistry, 2007). Some children have parents who see themselves as stewards of persons with their own emerging individuality, and not as little replicas of their elders. Others, without the benefit of conscious parenting in childhood, may only become attuned to their true nature later in life by mentors, healers, or spiritual teachers who see specific emergent qualities in a person never recognized before.

InnerView practitioners begin with the essential value of a person who is worthy by virtue of belonging to humanity. We begin any psychological exploration at the base camp of self-worth. The 4Fold Path map illustrates the basic geography of consciousness to navigate (Figure 4.1). Worth, in this case, is not a result of personality traits but is intrinsic to personhood. It does not depend solely on the efforts made to overcome painful legacies of the past. It does not need to be earned. One's value is not a result of working on oneself; it is presupposed. A person's value is already present before any course of therapy begins.

The nature of the ego is to earn its worth by accumulating the goods of life. For the soul it is the reverse. The soul reveals its worth through self-giving. For this reason, the InnerView approach makes the innermost nature of the person the starting point, rather than the end point of the therapeutic process (O'Hanlon et al., 2003). The analogy of the Russian nesting dolls represents both directions of therapeutic interventions:

outside-in (whereby the dolls are successfully unpacked until an irreducible one remains), and inside-out (like taking an X-ray of the intrapsychic realm to know how to realign the outer dolls with the innermost one). InnerView is an inside-out model, trusting the outgrowth of the core Self.

The Compassionate Gaze

Bringing a steady gaze to bear on the true Self of a person calls for an unconditionally loving observer, a witness who serves as an undistorted mirror of the client's true nature. It is a transition mirror for those at the outset of the inner journey who initially need the positive reflection to recognize it in themselves. The mirroring is a stage in the process of settling into the seat of personhood which informs, or rather, out-forms, the rest of the Russian doll personas surrounding it. The mirroring serves, at first, to affirm the natural shape of one's nature without the other layers of a constructed persona. It is mirroring that may not have been received in childhood, and so may take time to internalize. Once the positive perception is internalized it becomes self-validating. The burden of managing self-worth through external perceptions and judgments can then be lifted. In conflict situations, one can be inwardly free from the projections of others needing a bad guy in their story. The locus of meaning shifts from the terrain of external criteria (what other people think) to the landscape of creative manifestation (what we choose to bring into the world based on our own values).

The Matryoshka Method provides an alternative to the tendency of the medical model to probe for pathology. Imagine the smallest, innermost doll as imbued with the essential core goodness available to everyone. It is not good as opposed to bad, since human nature contains both. It is the goodness of our very existence, as an ontological foundation which can be trusted. Furthermore, if one could open the metaphorical core doll it would not be solid. It would be infinitely spacious, and inside of it would exist the source of all creative potentiality. Starting there changes our vision of a person. A true person, in the InnerView vision, is more like a portal for human possibilities than a product of social conditioning. Life-giving qualities are being expressed in and through each of us. We do not have to make something of ourselves to be of value. The best of life wants to be lived *through* each person in unique ways. Identity does not have to be settled once and for all. We can safely surrender to the flux of life. Opening to this more spacious sense of Self allows each individual to be in touch with their unique way of belonging to life.

Aligning the Layers

With this sense of Self, the other Russian doll layers can be built up more congruently, by realigning one's roles in the world, with the essential needs, values, and intentions of the core Russian doll. This ideally replaces the defence mechanisms developed to safeguard the self, with a translucent, free-flowing interplay between inner and outer worlds. The Matryoshka Method involves the faith it takes to seek with the soul and see with the heart. It is a simple concept, but a dramatic paradigm shift, like realizing the earth revolves around the sun rather than the converse. It begins with witnessing the inherent worth of the person and follows the 4Fold Path to restore the full presence, essence, and inner guidance of an individual. Life priorities are clarified accordingly. When life begins and ends with soul, it allows for a vision of original innocence, no matter how disordered its ego expression. When we are on a soul journey as well as a life path, then as Rainer Maria Rilke wrote: "We are born, so to speak, provisionally, it doesn't matter where. It is only gradually that we compose within ourselves our true place of origin so that we may be born there retrospectively and each day more definitely" (Mason, 2011).

One way or the other we are like Russian nesting dolls. The question is how congruently these dolls line up within us. In the therapeutic environment, each of the dolls represents a story the client is telling themselves about their life predicament. One of the ways the story becomes problematic is when a client thinks it is the definitive one, and the only source of self-concept they can have. It is associated with being a victim of circumstances. The emotional tendency is to contract around the story rather than expand on it. Rather than being perceived as just one layer of the whole person, the filter of the story leads the client to believe that there is only one part to play. To the extent that we identify with one of the dolls to the exclusion of the rest, especially the innermost one, a sense of one's full identity is limited.

The innermost doll or soul of the person represents what is of deepest value. It is self-knowledge not subject to the storylines of ego. When we are out of touch with this foundation, the outer dolls usurp that value like counterfeits pretending to be the real thing. When it comes to the constructed self, there are layers of these personas supported by the social context and the narrative of one's role in it. Identifying strongly with any of them can leave an individual feeling beside themselves with anxiety, depression, or the malaise of meaninglessness. The story of self when approached from the outside-in and animated by ego is based on the fear and limitations of the cover-up job represented by our outermost Russian dolls. It is also a way to safeguard the innermost doll from abuse experienced in childhood. The problem is that the longer the core doll stays in hiding or covered up by other personas, the more it reinforces the felt risks of exposure.

The Matryoshka Method has much in common with inner child dynamics and the therapeutic approach of reparenting oneself. Most inner child work involves revisiting powerless feelings of the past to process emotional wounds from an empowered adult position. Psychologically, that takes someone out of the victim position. Spiritually, we work with past stages of life in the awareness that both light and dark, positive and negative elements coexist in human nature. What harms us can also heal us. Spiritual work highlights the innocence, virtue, and light of the soul revealed in contrast to the self-image associated with ego damage. However, when ego identification predominates (outer Russian dolls) there is the fear that those shells will crack and expose more brokenness, down to the utter emptiness at the bottom of the constructed personality. When the inner child cries, "I'm scared, I'm vulnerable. I don't know how to survive on my own," it takes soul strength to counteract such ego dissolution. For some, that comes from a restored inner parent image. For others, it comes from trusting the immutable ground of Being, that which is called God in religious circles.

The Nature of Symptoms

For persons who cannot presuppose the existence of the innermost doll, the fear of facing the inner void when outer dolls are disassembled may seem utterly intolerable. That is when addictions enter the picture, as if the compensating Russian doll is saying, "I'm fine as long as I have my drink or drug of choice; as long as I'm shopping or working or gambling or in a gratifying relationship". When those strategies are exposed as safeguards against the pain of being unreal in relation to self and others, another Russian doll seeks relief from it all. Yet in turn, even the brokenness can be a safeguarding mechanism, the cover-up job of this damaged Russian doll saying, "I'm wounded and broken. I need to be fixed and that takes intensive therapy". However, it does not mean the therapy-wise Russian doll is ready to take her inner-view further. In the name of processing emotional pain, she may be treated in terms of a clinical condition and never gain access to a felt sense of the essential self.

The premise of The Matryoshka Method is that the foundation for human nature is good. We are not on trial for existing and if we were, we would be declared innocent. Therefore, the InnerView practitioner trusts that any distortions of one's true nature is just that and can serve as clues to the redeeming qualities seeking to be expressed through a person. What clinicians recognize as symptoms of a neurosis or personality disorder, the InnerView approach acknowledges as well. We are clear-sighted about the twists and turns of psychological malaise. Yet such disorders are still viewed as counterfeit versions of authentic personhood. The essential qualities accessible through the openheartedness of the innermost doll are still there to be elicited and put into service as curative factors. We hold the vision of that healing as a working hypothesis.

Personal and collective experiences of life shape one's way of being in the world. All lives have their setbacks and sadness. Emotional scars, family dysfunction, social chaos, and community upheaval are all real and have an immeasurable impact on the individual. We respect the problem-saturated Russian dolls, the ones guarding and protecting the gifts of the innermost one, contained and hidden within the outer layers. When one's connection with the innermost doll or true self is restored, professional guidance focuses on finding the most congruent expressions of it in the world. Based on intrinsic psychospiritual values, InnerView practitioners evoke qualities needed to rise to the challenges of life.

The Role of Therapy

Starting with qualities emerging from within the innermost doll, we move back through outer layers of identity, completing the set of nesting dolls. It is an expansive process, which counteracts the contractions of self-centeredness and encourages living in a bigger story. While problems and pain expose the emptiness within successive layers of false selves, we build up the true self. This is done by focusing on the underlying values and fullness of being which permeate the essence of a person. Instead of analysing the components of mental illness and offering antidotes for healthy coping, we expand the capacity to integrate all the contradictory parts into a meaningful whole in which all of selfhood is embraced. Intending to treat a person is about relieving symptoms. Trying to cure them is about removing the disease. True healing involves the whole person, to foster their growth beyond what holds them back. When the vision and values of the soul are restored, then psychological impediments can be addressed, emotional barriers overcome, and dysfunctional patterns broken. As one client said, "It was like a light coming on in a dark room, and suddenly I could see all the furniture I had been tripping over".

Most psychotherapeutic interventions are directed towards the goals of healthier self-esteem and more effective relationships. John Welwood differentiates that approach from the more inclusive one. "Psychological work focuses more on what has gone wrong: how we have been wounded in our relations with others and how to go about addressing that. Spiritual work focuses more on what is intrinsically right: how we have infinite resources at the core of our nature that we can cultivate in order to live more expansively" (Welwood, 2002). The ego is naturally interested in basic self-sustaining needs: security and survival, affection and esteem, control and power (Keating, Thiemann, & Pagels, 1999). However, spiritual growth is about transformation of consciousness supporting an ever-evolving Self that puts ego in perspective. From the soul's point of view, the priority is personal and collective evolution. Esteem is achieved through self-giving. The ego's need is to get what it wants. Yet ego strength is paradoxically needed for the courage it takes to relinquish control through spiritual surrender.

Conventional coaching and therapy typically lead from problems to solutions, powerlessness to personal agency, and groundlessness to stability. Psychospiritual guidance includes those outcomes while reframing them in service of self-transcending values. The synergy of spiritually integrated psychotherapy takes place when emotional issues are perceived as necessary catalysts for soul growth. Every time we choose connection over projection, transparency over strategy, vulnerability over power, and intentionality over opportunism, we are choosing soul over ego. Healthy functioning in terms of soul strength is necessary to contain the tensions of life (Figure 4.1). Where there are divisive ego interests, the soul has the capacity to hold the wholeness of being and forge a new synthesis from the competing dualities.

When traditional clinical protocols are applied to therapy, treating mental illness can paradoxically entrain the patient to remain in a problem-saturated state of mind. It is natural when people are hurting to want to find out what has gone wrong and make it right. When it is a matter of physical infection, for example, the medical model is applied by concentrating on the diseased area in order to examine and disinfect it, before providing the appropriate remedy. There are some parallels to emotional healing, yet unlike emotional wounds, the patient's personality is not shaped around the reaction to a physical injury (unless that is indeed part of their psychology).

Focusing on past traumatic events as the locus of investigation can inadvertently lead practitioners to view emotional woundedness as the main obstacle to full functioning. It sends the message that a person's underlying unhealthy core has diverted normal development. Addressing it is a long-term proposition, mired in methods of uncovering specific pathology, accomplished by peeling back layer after layer of the personality, searching for the origins of personal brokenness. This approach is at risk of becoming "woundology" whereby the eventual diagnosis becomes a badge of honour for psychological warriors who are survivors of trauma and victims of its consequences (Myss, 2004).

This is not to discount the value in knowing what set the stage for someone's current issues, especially when the role for which they were typecast in the dramas of the past can be re-authored in the present (Epston & White, 1994). Yet we do not want to lose sight of the whole person behind the partial problem, or the resilient soul subject to sustained defilement. There is something about the human person that remains intact even when the personality is shattered (Frankl, 2011). From the InnerView point of view, the person is a creative self-determining process rather than a product of past experiences.

The outside-in approach involves working through layers of psychological pain, using the onion skins metaphor in the name of uncovering the primal pain often associated with early trauma. There are definite historical sources of present problems, and history does tend to repeat itself both personally and collectively. However psychological pain unfortunately feeds upon itself in self-perpetuating ways, especially when it becomes the primary focus of attention. This is what Eckhart Tolle describes as the pain-body (Tolle, 2018). The emotional energy takes on a life of its own. To assuage this pain, traditional therapy is dedicated to uncovering repressed sources of present dysfunction. In the end, it helps clients disidentify with those underlying conditions by raising conscious awareness of how they can make different choices – internally and externally. Given this goal, what if we started with what is right and whole and good about a person, and build them up from there rather than breaking down the issues into pathological components?

Understanding Injury

The Matryoshka Method does not exempt anyone from painful life situations. Yet personal troubles are viewed from a different vantage point, that of the compassionate witness. Sometimes all it takes to release a burden is the validating gaze of unconditional acceptance. From that perspective self-defeating patterns, no matter how tight their grip, are viewed as distortions of a person's deepest truth. Given steady support of that truth, problems begin to look like catalysts for growth. The balance of attention shifts from what a person does *not* want to what they *do* want. Apparent misfortunes take on new meaning. As a client once said, "I now value as gift what I otherwise would experience as injury". Through the process of reframing, this client came to understand that what was happening *to* her could equally be viewed as happening *for* her. The Matryoshka Method can help clients realize it is not about what is going against them in life; it is what they can discover about themselves even under the most challenging of circumstances. Looking outward from the vantage point of the indomitable innermost doll, we can see everything from the flip side of the problem. As Albert Camus described it: "In the midst of winter, I found there was, within me, an invincible summer" (Camus, 1995).

InnerView guidance addresses emotional wounds, yet it does so in the context of healing images and redemptive experiences. The focus is on the shape life takes in the present, enabling the individual to live their truth and fulfil their goals. Clients are encouraged to see themselves as potentially self-actualizing rather than determined by damage from the past or defined by the judgments of others (Maslow, 1973). Past abuse can leave people feeling as if something is fundamentally wrong with them. The innermost Russian doll represents the essence of what is right with them, the inviolable soul. An InnerView assessment delves deeply into strengths and resources which motivate a client to move forward in the direction of their life purpose. Sources of discouragement are clues to the client's needs and values – pointing out unmet needs and unlived values. Problems appear insurmountable when they are in the foreground of attention. When we elicit essential qualities associated with the innermost Russian doll (e.g., courage, trust, loving-kindness) their place in the foreground of awareness allows problems to recede into the background, thereby loosening their grip.

Potential for Growth

Layers of personality are the outgrowth of an originally intact self, like the oak that grows from the acorn. That perspective supports confidence in one's potential. Believing all living beings have a built-in developmental destiny also undergirds healing and promotes further personal evolution (Hillman, 2017). To that end, InnerView guidance reframes previously troublesome elements of personality in terms of self-expansion, whereby soul strengths are brought to the fore as a result of painful past experiences. We look for the congruence of equal and opposite forces in character formation (Brooks, 2016; Crawford, 2016). It is a dialectical model of human development. Forgiveness emerges from a context of betrayal. Faith is found in the face of fear. Mercy is a response to judgement. Simplicity an answer to drama. Stillness implies busyness, nonattachment offsets disappointment, mindfulness an antidote to habitual reactions, intimacy juxtaposed with isolation, and loving-kindness is applied to aggression (Muller, 2002).

As applied by all helping professionals (coaches, counsellors, therapists, spiritual directors), InnerView seeks to narrow the gap between soul knowledge and the outer expression of it through social personas. InnerView practitioners use the skills of attunement and ongoing calibration, to align the soul with the rest of the personality in a consistent way. We hold the vision of the client's potential for healing. Along the way, we make room for the emotional wound and original wholeness to coexist. This increases the capacity for duo consciousness of the universal human predicament (Stanley, 2019). The thirteenth century Sufi master and poet, Jalaluddin Rumi, understood that although our human nature is fundamentally flawed, conscious awareness of the spiritual dimension is not: "Half of any person is wrong and weak and off the path. Half! The other half is dancing and swimming and flying in the Invisible Joy" (Jalal al Din & Barks, 2004).

The InnerView practitioner is one who helps find the crux of transformation and the call of metanoia in any life circumstance. The difference between a piece of black coal and a priceless diamond is how much pressure it has endured, as if withstanding the ordeal involves not doubting its destiny. A client could have good reasons to feel rejected and unworthy. Yet such negative conclusions imply their opposites, belonging and esteem, realities illuminated by the darkness of their felt absence. InnerView practitioners know from experience that clients can grow where they are planted. As dark and lonely, and buried in the backyards of life as a person may feel, we believe they are still divinely seeded for soul growth.

References

Benner, A. D., & Mistry, R. S. (2007). Congruence of mother and teacher educational expectations and low-income youth's academic competence. *Journal of Educational Psychology, 99*(1), 140–153. https://doi.org/10.1037/0022-0663.99.1.140

Brooks, D. (2016). *The road to character.* London: Penguin Books.

Camus, A. (1995). Retour de Tipasa. In *Summer.* London: Penguin Books.

Crawford, M. B. (2016). *The world beyond your head: On becoming an individual in an age of distraction.* Toronto, ON: Penguin Books.

DeShazer, S., Dolan, Y. M., & Korman, H. (2012). *More than miracles: The state of the art of solution-focused brief therapy.* London: Routledge.

Epston, D., & White, M. (1994). *Experience, contradiction, narrative & imagination: Selected papers of David Epston & Michael White, 1989–1991.* Adelaide, SA: Dulwich Centre Publications.

Frankl, V. E. (2011). *Man's search for ultimate meaning.* London: Rider.

Hillman, J. (2017). *The soul's code: In search of character and calling.* New York, NY: Ballantine.

Jalāl al Din, R., & Barks, C. (2004). *The essential Rumi: New expanded edition.* San Francisco, CA: Harper.

Keating, T., Thiemann, R. F., & Pagels, E. (1999). *The human condition: Contemplation and transformation.* New York, NY: Paulist Press.

MacKinnon, R. A., & Michels, R. (1971). *The psychiatric interview in clinical practice.* Philadelphia, PA: Saunders.

Maslow, A. H. (1973). *Dominance, self-esteem, self-actualization: Germinal papers of A.H. Maslow* (R. J. Lowry, Ed.). Monterey, CA: Brooks/Cole.

Mason, E. C. (2011). *Rilke, Europe, and the English-speaking world.* Cambridge: Cambridge University Press.

Merton, T. (2014). *Conjectures of a guilty bystander.* Garden City, NY: Image Books.

Muller, W. (2002). *Legacy of the heart: The spiritual advantages of a painful childhood.* New York, NY: Simon & Schuster.

Myss, C. M. (2004). *Anatomy of the spirit, and why people don't heal and how they can.* New York, NY: Gramercy Books.

O'Hanlon, W. H., Rowan, T., & Rowan, T. (2003). *Solution-oriented therapy for chronic and severe mental illness.* New York, NY: Norton.

Stanley, C. (2019). *Evolutionary leap: Colin Wilson on psychology.* London: Routledge.

Tolle, E. (2018). *The power of now: A guide to spiritual enlightenment.* Sydney: Hachette.

Welwood, J. (2002). *Toward a psychology of awakening: Buddhism, psychotherapy, and the path of personal and spiritual transformation.* Boston, MA: Shambhala.

6 InnerView Attunement

The Healing Bond in Therapeutic Practice

Attunement is the process whereby the consciousness of the practitioner influences the client beyond the content of their conversation (Erickson & Rosen, 1991). It extends the empathic bond of the rapport-building stage to mutual inner connection. It creates an intuitive alliance. A synchrony emerges between practitioner and client. That alignment is not limited to the shared content of the therapeutic sessions. It is a form of mental and emotional resonance based on the energetic interchange between persons (May, 1989). Lionel Corbett understands attunement as a shared experience: "While one can think of empathy in terms of limbic system resonance and the countertransference, these approaches do not take into account the spiritual importance of affective attunement. Shared affective states are important because they remind us that we are not separate entities – we participate in the same field of consciousness" (Corbett, 2015).

For attunement to take place, the practitioner must consciously maintain mindful awareness of the gap between the client's present struggle and the vision of healing needed to resolve it. This level of containment invokes the advanced skill of double awareness (Stanley, 2019). All therapists practice some form of dual attention to the content of client stories and to the overall process of therapeutic movement. The kind of double awareness facilitating attunement, however, involves "identification of subjective and objective resulting in a new condition which transcends them both" (May, 1989). In practice, this means the practitioner both emotionally identifies with the client's predicament and understands it dispassionately. In the practitioner's presence, the client experiences what it feels like to embody this dialectic. When attunement is effective, the client is subliminally invited to recover split-off aspects of themselves, as the practitioner enters their suffering without the struggle, and participates in their fractured sense of self without the self-division. This is congruent with the InnerView concept of the crossroads, where the wholeness of persons can coexist with their emotional wounds (Yaphe & Speyer, 2010).

Empathy and Dramatic Art

We can reach any person from within ourselves. The cathartic power of art is evidence of how empathy can extend to a fiction, as we identify with the experience of a character on stage or screen. While watching a good play or movie, we are taken out of ourselves and into the emotional experience of others. A powerful drama class exercise involves simply holding eye contact with a partner for a few minutes, prior to closing our eyes and taking in the presence of the other while being a curious observer of what arises in our awareness, without judging it. Subsequent debriefing of the exercise shows how real mental contact or pure heart connection can occur in the absence of any other input or agenda. Similarly, in the helping relationship at its best, what emerges between persons is greater than the sum of the parts and becomes a shared transmission or form of psychic transference (May, 1989).

To this end, the InnerView practitioner applies a kind of method acting in which any emotional associations the actor may share with the experience of his character are temporarily internalized. While remaining conscious of the nature and purpose of each scene, the method actor finds ways to identify with the essential personality traits of the character they are in effect, channelling. The therapeutic equivalent of this occurs when the practitioner enters the world view of the client and forms a bond on that basis. At the same time, we are also attuning the client to our consciousness which, when this is emulated by the client, begins to allow for different psychological plot lines. When a client feels trapped in a point of view which does not serve them, it is the attunement, not the analysis, which eventually leads the way out. The practitioner can fearlessly inhabit the room of limited options where it feels like the walls are closing in. Yet we can also stand in the doorway, offering a hand, ready to walk out into "the high meadows" with the client. In the words of Rumi:

> Don't be addicted to subtle discussions
> tying and untying knots, posing difficulties
> that then you resolve . . . .
> Remember how it feels to sail the mountain air
> and smell the sweetness of the high meadows.
> (Rumi & Barks, 2004)

Double Awareness

An effective therapeutic relationship depends on this capacity for entering another's inner world while steadily holding the space for remedial progress to be made. Double awareness (Stanley, 2019) is a way to sustain the creative tensions experienced by the person being attuned. Mature presence of mind is needed to balance subjective and objective points of view, thereby containing life's contradictions (Figure 4.2). Setting out to support the optimal functioning of the client in the world is useful yet sets the bar low. In seeking to narrow the gap between what is imagined in the inner world and what is manifested in the outer world, both realities need equal attention.

The importance of empathy in the therapeutic relationship has been well-documented (Kim, 2018). No client will truly consider any significant change in perspective or behaviour without first feeling completely accepted in their unhealed condition. The necessary glare of the assessment phase occurs when the practitioner brings the full scope of their clinical expertise to bear on the cause of the problematic core issue. Attunement, on the other hand, is the quality that allows us to relate to the presenting person, aside from the diagnosed issue. We affirm their fundamental human value. That is the unwavering gaze of encouragement.

A therapist in supervision, realizing the value of attunement, describes his experience as follows:

> More and more I understand that the context of each and every client includes the desire to move towards the best of who-they-are no matter what shape their pain is taking. The fact that a person struggles with a particular issue indicates that it is viewed in contradistinction to the best of who-they-are. In reaching for and relating to the best of who-they-are, it connects me with the best of who-I-am. I wonder . . . and suspect . . . that in being connected to my own essence it naturally leads clients to connect with their own. I recently read that what happens in the presence of those with extraordinary healing powers is that they clearly recognize and focus on the essence of others and, in so doing, everything that is not a part of that essence simply falls away or dissolves.
>
> (Peter Kerby, personal communication)

Attunement in Therapy

Attunement happens whenever we authentically relate to the essential beingness of the other while bracketing any diagnostic categories we have in mind which would objectify them. It is the way we are loved into living from our genuine nature. In therapy, attunement emphasizes the all-embracing gaze, while clearly acknowledging emotional wounds. For example, without minimizing the fallout from past abuse, attunement to client resiliency would implicitly send the following message in a therapy session.

You may have developed compensating qualities that originally helped you to survive childhood abuse. When you reclaim yourself in the present, those same qualities can be modified to support yourself and others. Hyper-vigilance at the time, for example, could become the gift of being able to offer your full attention in the present. The abuse may have also led you to doubt your worth. As an adult survivor capable of personal agency, you can choose to trust your innate value and exercise the gifts originally developed to ward off harm, much like inventions originating during wartime are later adapted for widespread societal use.

When practising the art and craft of helping, practitioners *themselves* are the tools of the trade. This involves bearing many creative tensions within oneself during a session, while remaining personable and at ease in the client's company. Just as the ballet dancer conveys through the body what is beyond the body, the presence and emotional demeanour of the practitioner speaks to the client beyond the words exchanged in a session. Words can be mere counselling clichés if they do not reflect genuine personal qualities (acceptance, patience, kindliness) demonstrated by the practitioner. Along with employing accepted therapeutic interventions, it is the therapist's state of mind and heart that can have the greatest influence.

Genuine engagement with the other person can produce an energetic third effect, with a life of its own transcending the two participants. As Carl Jung describes it, "The meeting of two personalities is like the contact of two chemical substances; if there is any reaction, both are transformed" (Jung, Dell, & Baynes, 2017). That psychospiritual atmosphere in the room works both ways, affecting the self-awareness of each person. The practitioner therefore needs the inner strength to sustain the hope of healing while under pressure from the client's legacy of discouragement, and psychic resistance to the healing synergy. When the attunement is effective, the true personhood of the client will emerge over time, drawn out into the open by the quality of consciousness resulting from the practitioner's own soul work. As healers, some of the emotional equanimity we transmit comes from the way we face the ambiguities of our own lives. To the extent we have done our own shadow work, emotional darkness is not countered with facile spiritual light. Lest this sound daunting, it does not mean the InnerView practitioner has to be a perfect person to qualify for having such an influence. Yet there is no substitute for genuineness. Former psychologist turned spiritual teacher, Ram Dass, critiques the false professional warmth that keeps relationships sterile and clients distant from professional helpers when he writes, "Perhaps the strategy for dealing with suffering most familiar in our helping institutions is that of 'professional warmth'. Like pity, it's a stance to keep our distance" (Ram & Gorman, 1989).

Being fully present in a counselling session is not as straightforward as it sounds. It involves paying dual attention to a number of elements. While present to the here-and-now encounter and listening attentively to the client's story, there needs to be a simultaneous witness in effect, dispassionately observing the drama without becoming too absorbed by it. As we closely follow descriptions of the client's struggle, we need to keep our distance from it, yet not the self-protective distance Ram Dass critiques. While seeing through a client's character armour, we also see them through their predicament. While alert to limiting beliefs, we foster freedom of choice. While we do what we can to relieve client distress, we do so with minimal attachment to the role of helper. Though we may acutely feel the social injustice of a client's life situation, it is not our job to fix anything. It is our job to attune clients to their own sense of effective personal agency.

The challenge lies in maintaining double awareness of the tensions within the client's personality as well those invoked or to be found in our own. By means of active listening and mindful witnessing, we fully attend to the client's story while temporarily bracketing any interpretations springing to mind. Empathy must always precede education. It is only when attuned to the client's emotional tone and perceptual frequency that we will be able to intuitively discern what form of guidance will most benefit them. C.G. Jung advises, "Learn your theories well, but put them aside when you touch the miracle of the living soul" (Jung, Baynes, & Baynes, 2008). It takes humility to work from the inside-out and not impose a preset therapeutic agenda on the process of soul work. We can keep the 4Fold Path map in mind, however, to locate where clients are starting from and moving towards on their developmental journey (Figure 4.1).

Through identification with the practitioner's openhearted demeanour and positive mirroring, clients learn to work through their troublesome feelings with self-compassion. Attunement always comes with tacit permission to relax. It allows anxiety and depression room in the psyche to be allies of unmet needs, rather than mere debilitating conditions. It invites clients to work with, rather than resist, the wisdom of the symptoms when they honour them as such. For example, an understandable depth of sadness can devolve into clinical depression when in the name of upbeat well-being it is identified solely as a condition to be treated. There is a place for treating clinical depression as such in the mental health system, especially from a neurobiological point of view, when symptoms are severe. Yet even that form of treatment needs to be offset with respect for the soul work of clients, who may need to go through the "dark night of the soul" (Moore, 2005). Otherwise, well-intended clinical interventions may press for an adjustment to a life that the soul does not want. Therefore, our first responsibility as InnerView practitioners is to open the door to Rumi's "guest house", in which the gamut of human emotions is likened to honoured guests invited to make themselves at home. In Rumi's words:

> This being human is a guest house.
> Every morning a new arrival.
> A joy, a depression, a meanness,
> some momentary awareness comes
> As an unexpected visitor.
> Welcome and entertain them all!
>   (Rumi & Barks, 2004)

Unconditional Regard

The poet John Keats calls the unconditional and purely attentive capacity "negativity capability". As applied to therapy, it is the ability to suspend an agenda that could compromise curative factors. This involves doing our own ongoing shadow work to separate out subjective biases, subconscious blind spots, defences, countertransferences, unresolved personal complexes, culture-specific biases, social conditioning, family-of-origin triggers, and any forms of self-deception which might get in the way of being fully present to clients. To the extent our own psyche is cleared for duty this way, we will be able to relate in truly empathic ways. Carl Rogers describes empathy as

> entering the private perceptual world of the other and becoming thoroughly at home in it. It involves being sensitive, moment to moment, to the changing felt meanings which flow in this other person, to the fear or rage or tenderness or confusion or whatever he or she is experiencing.
>
>   (Rogers, 1975)

Rogers speaks of being a confident companion to the other person in their world.

While the clinical glare reveals what we need to know about the distortions of personality, the healing gaze affirms the person's inherent capacity to realize their true nature. Sometimes all it takes is being summoned by unfiltered attention to the quality of personhood underlying personality. An excerpt from a letter written by the Trappist monk, Benedict Vanier, to his mother Pauline describes this form of attunement in terms of her gift of pure presence. "Now", Vanier asks, "what exactly does this gift do? It identifies [others]. . . . You bring them out of their anonymity, you make them vibrate as persons, because you vibrate as a deeply personal being . . . you help to bring them out of [their anonymity] and their personhood comes into play because of the register of your presence" (Coady, 2015). When someone gives us their undivided attention and there is no agenda besides the authenticity of the encounter itself, it is a transformative experience. Cynthia Bourgeault describes the depth of such an encounter in her book *Mystical Hope* when as a young graduate student she met the founder of the Taizé Community, Frère Roger Schütz.

> He looked deeply into me and through me, into depths I never even knew were there. For the next thirty seconds, I had his full attention – perhaps the first time this had ever happened to me in my life, the first time I had ever experienced what it means to be unconditionally loved. I left that encounter with my heart overflowing with hope; by the following year I was baptized. And it was nothing he said – just the power of the way he was present, his complete transparency to love.
>
> (Bourgeault, 2001)

Consciousness precedes anything in it, any object of consciousness, including thought. The individual subjectivity we locate in our apparently separate minds has a substratum of awareness which we all have in common. It is often referred to as the unified field or ground of being. That which some call God is the source of unconditioned, formless consciousness, localized like beams of light emerging from a movie projector, taking form in the drama appearing on the screen. In this analogy, the client beginning therapy is like someone absorbed in, and identified with, the drama whereas the practitioner is consciously following the plot from the point of view of the audience. It takes unwavering faith to sustain the knowledge that we are not defined by our problems or flaws. Attunement allows for the realization that there is a backstage consciousness to access, a spacious awareness where human freedom is to be found, not bound by psychodynamics. By the very way we resonate with clients on a soul level, we are not just helping them cope but facilitating the flow of life-giving current capable of breaking through logjams in the psyche. As Rumi reminds us: "When

you do things from your soul, you feel a river moving in you, a joy. . . . /
Ask the way to the spring / Your living pieces will form a harmony"
(Rumi & Barks, 2004).

References

Bourgeault, C. (2001). *Mystical hope – Trusting in the mercy of God*. Cambridge, MA: Cowley Publications.

Coady, M. F. (2015). *Mercy within mercy: Georges and Pauline Vanier and the search for God*. London: Darton, Longman & Todd.

Corbett, L. (2015). *Sacred Cauldron: Psychotherapy as a spiritual practice*. Asheville, NC: Chiron Publications.

Erickson, M. H., & Rosen, S. (1991). *My voice will go with you: The teaching tales of Milton H. Erickson*. New York, NY: W.W. Norton.

Jung, C. G., Baynes, H. G., & Baynes, C. F. (2008). *Contributions to analytical psychology* (p. 361). Hong Kong: Hesperides Press.

Jung, C. G., Dell, W. S., & Baynes, C. F. (2017). *Modern man in search of a soul*. Eastford, CT: Martino Fine Books, 2017.

Kim, S. (2018). Therapist's empathy, attachment, and therapeutic alliance: Neurobiological perspective. *International Journal of Psychology & Behavior Analysis*, 4, 140. https://doi.org/10.1002/cpp.792.

May, R. (1989). *The art of counselling*. New York, NY: Gardner Press.

Moore, T. (2005). *Dark nights of the soul*. New York, NY: Avery.

Ram, D., & Gorman, P. (1989). *How can I help?: Emotional support and spiritual inspiration for those who care for others*. London: Rider.

Rogers, C. R. (1975). Empathic: An unappreciated way of being. *The Counseling Psychologist*, 5, 2–10. https://doi.org/10.1177/001100007500500202.

Rumi, J., & Barks, C. (2004). *The essential Rumi: New expanded edition*. San Francisco, CA: Harper.

Stanley, C. (2019). *Evolutionary leap: Colin Wilson on psychology*. London.: Routledge.

Yaphe, J., & Speyer, C. (2010). Using email to enrich counselor training and supervision. In K. Anthony, D. M. Nagel, & S. Goss (Eds.), *The use of technology in mental health: Applications, ethics and practice*. Springfield, IL: Charles C. Thomas.

7 The Principles in Practice
InnerView Applied by
Helping Professionals

Throughout this book we have presented the theoretical foundations of InnerView Guidance. In this chapter, we are privileged to present the stories of eight practitioners who describe how InnerView principles pertain to their professional lives. The stories of their unique professional paths and practices bring the theory to life and demonstrate how it can be applied in very different therapeutic environments. We hope this will provide readers with further insight into the value and scope of the model as reflected in these examples.

The eight firsthand accounts included here are linked with central themes covered in the preceding chapters. The first entry on applications in family medicine reflects the current clinical landscape and shows how medical training can be informed by the InnerView perspective. The second and third stories reveal how the platform of online counselling served as a testing ground for a very different view of clients. The next essay on sandplay therapy illustrates how issues are reframed when they become part of the archetypal process of soul work. The fifth practitioner reveals how elements of the 4Fold Path are congruent with spiritual direction. In the sixth piece, the essential principles of peacemaking and conflict resolution are compared with The Matryoshka Method. In the last two accounts, the nature of attunement is made more accessible through experiences of it by practitioners in different settings. All these contributions add up to InnerView having a wide range of applicability to the helping professions.

InnerView Applied to Family Medicine
John Yaphe

Family medicine has been enriched by many influences in the last half-century. InnerView Guidance is one of the models that has helped expand my own horizons. It provides a way to view patients as persons first. People come to doctors with life stories, cultural contexts, generational legacies, and strengths of character, all of which make clinical diagnosis just one part of the complete picture.

My personal and professional journey has taken me across three continents in a wide range of professional and academic contexts. I was trained initially in the scientific method at the medical school of McGill University in the 1970s. Teaching in psychiatry provided a grounding in psychodynamic approaches as well as information on the rapid developments in pharmacology. However, all of this took place in the classroom or hospital setting with little contact in the community outside the walls of the institution. There was no mention of the soul, or its expressions in art, religion, spirituality, or the universal human quest for meaning. Yet these forms of growth were always there, in the unwritten curriculum. They were expressed in the ways our patients spoke to us and in the ways that the best of our teachers responded to them.

In my family medicine training in Israel in the 1980s, I worked in farming villages, with cultures I had never previously encountered. I heard about life challenges that were not yet part of my clinical experience. The training program at that time was cross-fertilized by exciting new ideas from family therapy, medical anthropology, humanistic psychology, and narrative approaches. All this shaped my work beyond the biomedical model. The puzzle of discovering the right clinical diagnosis was often of secondary importance to learning the life story and assessing the inclusive self, embedded in a larger context. I learned to understand the extent of full personhood involving meaning and purpose. This is what InnerView calls living in a bigger story.

My practice was also shaped by sabbatical years in London, Ontario, and Oxford, England, exploring patient-centred care. Medical education became a process of personal and professional growth, rather than simply transmitting expertise. The union of quantitative and qualitative methods led to generating new knowledge, relevant to patients in community settings. I found value in hearing individual stories of how patients coped with illness. All this meant that the self-awareness of the clinician, teacher, and researcher was of great importance. To be a reflective practitioner means working from the inside-out, allowing for attunement with patient experience by touching upon how it resonates within oneself.

My current clinical practice involves international online counselling. I apply the principles of InnerView Guidance at the crossroads of where the client's journey in the outside world intersects with the quality of their inner life. I share these ideas with medical students, to enrich the curriculum of the social and psychological determinants of health. They also learn the importance of healing relationships based on underlying values. I participate in an online forum with other InnerView practitioners for the same reasons. The sharing of personal and professional challenges from the viewpoint of soul growth shows how far-reaching this path can be.

John Yaphe is a family physician with a special interest in counselling. He studied medicine in Canada and worked as a family doctor and as a teacher of family medicine in Israel for 27 years. He has published over 60 peer-reviewed scientific articles, including research in online counselling. He is currently Associate Professor at the School of Medicine of the University of Minho, in Braga, Portugal, where he teaches courses on psychological and social determinants of health. He has worked as an online counsellor for the past 16 years.

InnerView Applied to Online Counselling
Ralph Friesen

The remote community where I live in the Rocky Mountains of Canada is not that easy to visit. The nearest airport frequently cancels flights because of low cloud ceilings. In winter, heavy snowfalls can make the roads practically impassible. Two winters ago, when the power went out for several hours, my wife and I went to the neighbours and we gathered around their wood stove for warmth. Yet here in the mountains, I regularly met clients from all over the continent and beyond, without actual seeing or hearing them, in the early days of text-based online counselling.

When we meet a person face-to-face, whether physically present with them or via video, we form a quick impression, based on what we perceive of their whole demeanour. That impression is often filtered through our previous experience of apparently similar personality types. This also happens in the therapeutic relationship, on both sides. When the idea the client has of us is mainly a projection of their past relationships, it is called transference. When we see the client through our preconceptions or expectations, it is called countertransference. Obviously, both these effects interfere with a clear view of the real person. Even on the telephone, we make gut-level assessments based on what we sense about the quality of the other's voice, and any familiar resonance it may have for us.

When the meeting between practitioner and client happens solely via the written word (the back-and-forth of text-based exchanges) something remarkable takes place. With the static of visible personality traits removed from the communication channel a heart-to-heart, even soul-to-soul dialogue can take place. All we have is text on the screen, set there by a person who is invisible and inaudible to us. We are missing many of the cues we normally have when in each other's physical presence. Yet the absence is not a matter of something lacking in this context. It becomes a shared space for coauthoring a different story in service of the client's true self, free of how their outer persona might be perceived.

By applying the InnerView orientation to my practice, I gradually developed the capacity to engage clients in soul talk which points both psychology and spirituality toward what life wants from us, not just what we want out of life. It naturally changes the conversation from overcoming obstacles to well-being, to the old idea of how suffering can shape character when a person responds to it that way. I learned to zone in on what their life predicament had to say about where they were on their soul journey. The medium is conducive to entering the client's worldview while maintaining my own. The text-based format also allows the use of healing images from nature, metaphors, symbols, analogies, teaching stories, in short, anything that taps into the wellspring of the client's own creativity.

Online counselling is not seen as alternative as it used to be. And yet let us not lose sight of how miraculous it is. While the safety and containment of each of us on either side of our computers is not quite the same as gathering around a wood stove, the unique experience of non-local presence, that feeling of being alone together, brings it all back home.

Ralph Friesen is a marriage and family therapist, with degrees in English literature. He recently published *Dad, God, and Me*, a memoir/biography. See his website for more background: www.ralphfriesen.com/ Now retired, Ralph is also an amateur historian, with a focus on Mennonite history. He is the author of *Between Earth & Sky: Steinbach, the First 50 Years*, which won the Margaret McWilliams Award for excellence in local history, Manitoba. He is also the coauthor of an intergenerational family history, *Abraham S. Friesen, Steinbach Pioneer*. Ralph lives in Nelson, BC with his wife, Hannah.

InnerView Applied to Online Supervision
Cedric Speyer

In the spring of 2000, I pioneered an online counselling program in Canada on a large scale and with more scope than any of us in the helping professions had previously experienced online. We began with short-term, text-based cases, which was still relatively uncharted territory at that time. It necessitated new methods for both the primary practice and the quality assurance of training and supervision, also conducted mainly online. Equipped with short-term solution-oriented methods, and the old-fashioned art of letter-writing (via time-delayed web board exchanges) I found myself scouting ahead as a new path and practice unfolded. It led to the genesis of the model we now call InnerView Guidance.

In the space of a few years, our growing "e-team" completed thousands of cases and consistently received client feedback that confirmed the overall efficacy and value of the medium. Yet, in December 2007, in response to a feature on the success of our online service, the following letter to the editor appeared in *The Toronto Star*:

> E-therapy makes me uneasy. Online, (patients) can easily omit certain thoughts or feelings. The therapist does not have the advantage of examining body language and tone of voice. . . . It is much easier to distort the written word. Add mental illness to the mix, and you have a potentially dangerous situation.

Szymczak, P. (2007, December 8). E-therapy doesn't solve real problems. (Letter to the Editor). *The Toronto Star*.

Critics of online communication often dwell on the absence of nonverbal cues and thereby fail to appreciate how transparent some clients can be in text. Feelings about physical appearance, demeanor, and being on the spot in person were no longer a factor on either side. As a result of the disinhibiting effect of not being seen, clients tended to be more direct and self-disclosing in writing than face-to-face. The online practitioners, in turn, learned to read between the lines and pick up on the nuances of text-based cues. It felt like we had a window into the thought processes and emotional state of clients. With experience and the help of close supervision when needed, online practitioners developed the ability to read client exchanges more intuitively and respond in kind. We were discovering a new wavelength of interpersonal empathy unique to the modality. Text-based bonding is the term for the experience of telepresence, or nonlocal presence; the feeling of being with someone, albeit at a physical distance, in a computer-mediated relationship.

As a supervisor, I witnessed three main ways of relating to clients in writing. The least conducive to text-based bonding is writing *at* the presenting problem with informed commentary on the issue (which could be found in a blog or self-help article). An example would be teaching the client good communication habits without connecting from the heart oneself. The second level is writing *to* the issue, by focusing mainly on the content of the client's reported life situation, while suggesting possible coping methods (which can sound like an advice column). That could result in addressing a marital impasse, for instance, without attending to the pain of the person going through it. The third and most advanced approach to the online alliance is writing *with* the person behind the problem. Since the format of text-based counselling lends itself to psychoeducation, practitioners had to learn to avoid the trap of overdoing the didactic guidance. On the other hand, if they tried to emulate active listening and track ongoing instances of the problem, practitioners could end up being mere sounding boards. They needed to take the lead when writing back, without overloading the dialogue with a directive agenda. That balance was achieved by exploring and supporting what would motivate the client on their own terms.

The modality called for specialized skills in reading as well as writing. It helped that as a supervisor, I had a background in the creative arts, and not just counselling psychology. When we position ourselves as coauthors of a bigger story, it allows clients to approach the growing edge of what the soul wants under the circumstances. From that expanded perspective, they may find they have a heroic role to play in an otherwise intolerable life situation. We accomplish this by entering a shared narrative space from our side of the computer. When the client's story and the practitioner's layered reading of it coalesce, it leads to a creative synergy producing new possibilities. There is an energetic joining which is mutually felt. When we accompany a client to the crossroads and see them make a conscious choice of direction, ready to continue on their way without us by their side, and wave a heartfelt goodbye, it is easy to forget that we never actually met.

Cedric Speyer is a writer and Registered Psychotherapist. As a clinical supervisor, he developed the InnerView model and designed the 4Fold Path map depicting the sequences of soul work. Cedric pioneered online counselling on a large scale in Canada and helped establish its credibility, before cofounding InnerView Guidance International (IGI): https://innerviewguidance.com/.

InnerView Applied to Sandplay Therapy
Sheila Dorothy Smith

The InnerView framework describes psychological growth and integration as soul work, as sacred story. Images of quest, descent, crossroads, and transformation help us catch inklings about the process of soul work. These images are the currency of myth, ritual, poetry, legend, dreams, and alchemy. They are also terms of the InnerView paradigm. As a teacher and psychotherapist having offered Sandplay both in the school and in the therapy room, I have witnessed the metaphors of soul journey, as they are made visible in sandtrays, retold in stories and embodied in the play of children and adults. As a participant in a personal Sandplay process I have experienced their resonance.

In Sandplay, a bridge, boat, serpent, or castle can be manoeuvred within a physical terrain of mountain, desert, river, or cave. The sandpicture that emerges holds up a mirror to the sandplayer's *inner view*; it is the interior landscape made manifest. Because it bypasses the ego's agenda and the limitations of the spoken word – both of which can be impediments to inner work – Sandplay can invite the hero's journey. It is a form of active imagination.

I offer the following stories from my practice with gratitude and with respect to the two whose inner work is referenced here:

A middle-aged woman places in the sand tray a thicket of dry sticks. It dominates the landscape, bisecting it diagonally. On one side is a donkey laden with cooking pots, a dragon, and a prospector; on the other side rests a white porcelain tea set. The sandpicture brings to mind the contrast between a Victorian parlour and an outpost saloon. When a feather floats down from the thicket the woman becomes frustrated: "I feel like saying f– – –!" she says. "It won't do what I want it to!" In the outer world this person is facing multiple, severe life challenges. In the inner world she is living the divided landscape. The therapist informed by the InnerView perspective is a guide at the crossroads, aware that the feather floating down from the thicket could signal a third alternative; one available at the intersection of the vertical (spiritual) dimension and her horizontal (worldly) path. Perhaps what appears to be a stalemate could be the very point of entry to the bigger story.

A preadolescent boy comes to therapy when he has begun to self-harm. He works in mediums of clay and sand to project and embody his sense of powerlessness, his aggrieved relationship with a sibling, and the cognitive distortions he holds about self-sacrifice. Eventually, with the aid of vast swathes of dialogue he has memorized, he introduces his personal mentors – the mythic dragon-slaying heroes of his favourite movies. Six months after beginning the process, he creates a new sandpicture. A fence bisects the landscape. At the very centre, a boy figure stands wide-armed at a gate. "This is me at the gate," he explains. "I'm saying, 'Welcome to Glory!'" He closes the gate slowly and adds, "The gate used to be shut like this". He opens it again: "But – the boy chooses to open it!" In InnerView terms, "The choice of whether to expand or contract in response to life predicaments" is made, and the choice is expansion.

InnerView re-envisions life stories as soul journeys. A surprise feather falling from a hedge of dry sticks, a gate opening to a field called Glory: these are intimations of the wonder and the trueness of that vision.

Sheila Dorothy Smith is a registered psychotherapist in Ontario currently maintaining a part-time private practice in Jungian sandplay and expressive play therapy. She is the author of *Sandtray Play and Storymaking:*

A Hands-On Approach to Build Academic, Social Emotional and Skills in Mainstream and Special Education (Jessica Kingsley Press, 2012) and contributed to *The Routledge International Handbook of Sandplay Therapy* (Routledge, 2017). Sheila proposes a model for embedding sandtray play within the language arts curriculum, a model she developed during her years as a Special Education teacher in the elementary school system in Ontario, Canada.

InnerView Applied to Spiritual Direction
Maria Eusebia da Silva

Some time ago I dreamed I was walking up a hill and it was a tremendous struggle to put one foot in front of the other. Suddenly I felt myself being lifted a few inches off the ground by a gentle wind and carried up the hill. The experience of being carried by the wind left me feeling joyful, exuberant. The dream captured both the feeling of arduous effort and the unearned grace I experience when engaged in various forms of spiritual care.

As a spiritual director and retreat leader, I regularly turn to the Spiritual Exercises, a practical manual written by Ignatius of Loyola, the 16th-century mystic and founder of the Jesuit religious order. Ignatius developed the Exercises as a guide for spiritual directors who accompany others seeking to deepen their relationship with the divine. Through meditation (praying with words, images, and ideas) and contemplation (praying with scripture through feelings and imagination), Ignatius discovered that a *soul* (the spark of God in each person) aligns with the *Spirit* (God), moving past *ego* to free up the whole *self* (what Ignatius calls spiritual freedom).

In my work I find the 4Fold Path, with its compass points of full personhood to be a useful map. By using the guideposts of the Spirit (north), Soul (south), Psyche (east), and Ego (west), I guide the retreatant to a sense of how balanced or unbalanced they are in the big picture of their present situation. How close are they to the crux of the issue, or the central locus of their soul work? Similarly, using the language of my spiritual training, I help them consider how much spiritual freedom they are experiencing. Are they relying on a label from the outside world for self-definition? Or can they, like the Samaritan woman, described in the story below, find their true self in the encounter with the divine? For both director and retreatant, this journey is a mixture of work (prayer, deepening their connection with the divine) and grace (surrender, letting that relationship lead to further discernment).

In the gospel account of the woman at the well (John 4:1–42), the transformation that can happen over a long course of therapy is distilled in one encounter with Jesus. A woman comes to draw water from the town's well. That she comes alone and at the heat of midday suggest she is alienated from her community. There she meets Jesus who initiates a dialogue by asking her for water. During the ensuing conversation, Jesus awakens a thirst in her for something more than well water. Without judging her, Jesus reveals that he knows her history, yet it does not define her true nature. Surprisingly, he also reveals his true Self. The encounter is equivalent to the InnerView crossroads for her. At any time, the Samaritan woman could stop the conversation or walk away. She does not do either. As in my dream, she continues to make the effort, keeping the flow of dialogue going. Something shifts. She comes to realize that she is not defined by her cultural identity or previous marriages. She leaves behind her water jar to tell her world the news.

This brief healing encounter can be viewed as a microcosm of the main 4Fold Path sequence. Jesus is a *witness* to the social trappings masking her true self. By fully entering the shared *presence* at the well, the meeting is no longer between strangers separated by individual and collective identity. Jesus taps into the *essence* of her humanity through the unconditional relatedness he offers her. Her world has become larger. There is implicit *guidance* in the way she now views herself and her community. In this bible story, the Samaritan woman has experienced the kind of transformation that psychospiritual guidance offers.

Spiritual direction and therapy are alike in that both are a relationship between two people for the wellbeing of the retreatant or the client. Yet spiritual direction is relational in another sense, in that at its core it is about relationship with God. I am grateful that the psychospiritual approach of InnerView is congruent with my pastoral path and practice. It begins with viewing my own life challenges as opportunities for soul growth. That hopeful perspective extends to those I support when they find themselves at a crossroads on their journey of faith.

Maria Eusebia da Silva is a Registered Psychotherapist in Ontario, Canada. She has worked as a spiritual care practitioner in a variety of health care settings and in the community with individuals released from prison. She is engaged in the ministry of spiritual direction and leads retreats and workshops on spirituality. Maria cofounded InnerView Guidance International (IGI) and has contributed to the ongoing development of the InnerView model.

InnerView Applied to Conflict Transformation
Jessica Hawkins

Peacework, seen through the InnerView lens, involves more than conflict resolution interventions and third-party political strategies. It reintroduces the often-overlooked element of integrative soul work, which brings inner and outer worlds, as well as the individual and collective, into more harmonious alignment.

One of the first important lessons I learned in international peacework came in 2011, as I was escorting a Darfur-based rebel group to peace talks with the government of Sudan. To me, it seemed a hopeful and exciting time – there was finally going to be peace. When only seven of the nine men we expected arrived at the plane, I asked the leader about the missing two. He said, "Oh, they were shot in battle last night." What?! That didn't make sense to me. Weren't we in the middle of establishing peace?

I realized something that day and in the days that followed, as the world applauded and celebrated the signing of the Doha Peace Agreement. It is the shortsightedness of dealing with conflict superficially, on the transactional surface. Yes, the fighting might come to a mandated halt, at least as long as the terms last, but the energy of the conflict will endure and find other forms of expression. To work towards lasting social change, we must be willing to engage all layers of a given system, facilitating greater cohesion between them. This reminds me of The Matryoshka Method, with its realignment of the outer Russian dolls, congruent with the innermost one.

Moving into the intrapersonal sphere, such as that found in the therapeutic environment, we find similar oversights. Dominant approaches aimed at identifying the root causes of inner conflict focus predominantly on pathologies and the dysfunctions that ensue. Neuroscience shows us that the brain changes in response to experiences, for better or worse. Unfortunately, digging deeper into the damaging effects of conflict or trauma may be counterproductive, as it could unintentionally intensify emotional injuries. Interventions guided by the assumption that focusing on disorder will help bring about recovery are not only insufficient; in my view they are inconsistent with the primary aim of facilitating greater personal harmony and healing.

InnerView guidance provides not only a clinical philosophy, but also a framework for understanding a person's pathway through the psychospiritual realm. It holds the polarities of human experience within a greater whole and encourages practitioners to embrace the dialectic of conflict and peace. Instead of engaging in traditional root-cause analysis, InnerView guides conduct a root-core synthesis. By "seeking with the soul and seeing with the heart", conflict can be reframed as a portal, painful though it may be, to one's innermost values and purposes. It can act as an important signpost pointing towards what truly matters and reveal deep-seated needs and desires. In InnerView terms, it is "what the soul wants".

Peace, seen through this lens, can be understood as ever-present, embodied in the bedrock of our common humanity. Practitioners working at these levels can help expand both inner and outer horizons, by harnessing conflict and tapping into its creative potential. Conflict can be an impetus for deep and authentic transformation. Working with what constitutes the healthy person or community, can help both individuals and groups with the inner/outer congruence we call peace.

Jessica Hawkins holds a master's degree in peace and conflict Studies from the University of Innsbruck and is an accredited solution-focused practitioner and conflict coach. She specializes in solution-focused approaches to conflict transformation. As a former consultant to the United Nations, Jessica brings experience in peace and conflict work to InnerView guidance. She is a mother to a two-year-old and four-year-old, who teach her the true meaning of peace, and help to hone her skills in conflict transformation.

InnerView Applied to Intuitive Wellness Coaching
DeeAnna Nagel

A golden thread runs through the teachings of InnerView Guidance. It was hard for me to see myself until by holding onto that thread I found my way through the maze of psychological theories and could better help clients find a way out of their life impasses. My golden thread is intuitive wellness coaching. InnerView Guidance calls it attunement. As psychospiritual practitioners, it is the qualification we most need to trust. We are guides at the crossroads, regardless of our job title or specific vocation. Those of us informed by this approach are called to see with the heart and seek with the soul, which has not yet led to a new compendium of diagnostic criteria.

As a psychotherapist turned intuitive wellness coach, I always felt I was doing soul work until one day a supervisor described my work with clients as too "prescriptive" in the clinical sense of treating patients according to the *Diagnostic and Statistical Manual of Mental Disorders* (DSM). Upon reflection, I believe I became a licensed psychotherapist first and foremost to justify my natural intuitive gifts. I did not think intuitive work of any kind could stand on its own merit. In the moment I was told about my issue-based and therefore limited approach to therapy, I was more than taken aback. I was aghast; even I daresay, on the defensive.

Some time later, I realized how the culture of counselling and psychotherapy in the United States is largely based on avoiding litigation. Consequently, as a psychotherapist, however much I emphasized person-centred care in my practice, I continued to feel trapped in the medical morays of diagnosis and pathology: these are the necessities of the third-party payment system here in America. My work with clients was solid. I led with compassion. Yet over time, matching my dialogue with clients to case notes related to insurance forms felt increasingly oppressive to me.

Finally, after practising psychotherapy for fifteen years I chose to train as a wellness coach, which dovetailed with concurrent InnerView mentorship. I began to apply InnerView principles on my personal and professional path. This, in turn, influenced how I conceived of my vocation. Freed from the clinical checklists associated with my former role, I was able to stretch my intuitive aptitudes, connect more genuinely and engage more collaboratively with clients. Instead of probing for sources of emotional wounds, I focused on what is right in a person's life. When assessing, I began "above the wellness line" and kept the inclusive self in mind. That provided the benchmark for attunement when the issues clients brought to therapy revealed what was incongruent with their healthiest self.

I also learned to listen. Surprising, since listening skills are the prerequisite for any helping relationship. Yet, I now see that I did not really attend with my full presence until I was no longer bound by the self-serving aspects of the American medical model. My work became more heart-centred as I listened intuitively to others. Soul work allows for hearing with the third ear and letting the sixth sense into the coaching process. It is a way of knowing a person beyond what we can assess from what is spoken of in-session.

The energetic exchange between a client and an intuitive wellness coach is, at times, palpable. As I listen to their story, I intentionally tune into the subtle resonance underlying what is being shared. Often what the client needs to hear will emerge spontaneously, as a revelation to both of us. As one client described his struggle adjusting to a pending divorce, he told me he just could not imagine leaving the family home. When he said that, I visualized a carefully constructed bird's nest. At first, I thought of it simply as a metaphor that might validate his feeling of not wanting to make a go of it on his own. Yet I sensed more to the story. When I told him that the image of the bird's nest came to me, his face lit up. "Oh! Nests are not where birds roost – they are for keeping eggs and chicks in place." The client had the epiphany that his real need was to keep his children safe. Once assured of that, he would feel free to move on from the marriage.

Witnessing a client learn to trust their inner voice and reclaim themselves in that way, is one of the gifts of InnerView Guidance. Along the way, I have learned to not let go of my end of the golden thread. When it comes to clients who are in transition or upset by a life event, I trust that the best of my thread will be woven into the tapestry of their life as they journey forward, trusting their own intuitive guidance.

DeeAnna Nagel is a former psychotherapist turned intuitive wellness coach. She teaches coaches and therapists about alternative approaches to health and wellness, among other topics, and how to deliver these services ethically, whether in-person or via distance technology: https://havanawellnessstudio. com/. She is considered a thought leader in the fields of online therapy and coaching as well as distant healing. In addition to life and wellness coaching credentials, she is certified in aromatherapy and energy healing. DeeAnna is enrolled in a doctoral programme through SCA University of Theology and Spirituality (expected 4/2022) with a focus on spiritual direction.

InnerView Applied to Trauma Sensitive Yoga
Deborah McDermott

The holding of space is a sacred act and in that holding, another is free to simply *be*. The unconditional embrace of a person's present state creates a safe atmosphere for healing at their own pace. It allows nature to take its course. InnerView Guidance uses the term *attunement* for the energetic effects of trusting the helping relationship on this non-verbal, subliminal level. As a yoga therapist guiding trauma sensitive yoga experiences, it is congruent with my own practice.

For as long as I can remember, I have known my body has a natural wisdom of its own. Often this felt sense made more sense to me than what my head had to say about a life situation, with its competing points of view and reliance on analysis. When I was first drawn to yoga it was introduced to me as healthy exercise. Yet for me, it felt like a way of extending the conversation I was already having with my body. When I became a yoga teacher, I learned more about the healing that yoga practice offers on different levels. This led to further training as a yoga therapist and in that role, I came across many trauma survivors who felt stuck in unintegrated emotional states. When I discovered trauma sensitive yoga, it completely resonated with me. By privileging body-knowing over mental processing, I find it to be uniquely therapeutic for survivors of complex trauma.

Trauma Sensitive Yoga (TSY) is used in conjunction with traditional talk therapy, to help trauma survivors heal. The pain, confusion, and emotional challenges clients show up with are natural reactions to what they have gone through. It is evidence of their wholeness seeking to be restored, not of their brokenness. InnerView describes attunement as allowing the client's woundedness and wholeness to coexist. It attends to the person, not a diagnosis. It shifts the focus of the work from fixing (what is broken) to connecting (with what is naturally integrative). What InnerView and TSY have in common is a deep respect for the true nature of persons.

Yoga therapy and especially trauma sensitive yoga are very different from what most people think of as a yoga class. Survivors of complex trauma almost universally have a negative, even hateful relationship with their own bodies. They tend to push away the experiences of their bodies. TSY guides clients to interocept (bring conscious awareness to body sensation), and then make choices about what they perceive on a somatic level. Clients are repeatedly invited to make free choices: arms up, arms to the side, not moving the arms at all; bending the knee or not bending the knee; moving with the breath or holding a position and breathing in it, etc. It is normal in a TSY class to see everyone doing something a little (or a lot) differently. The class is an experience of learning how to feel (embody) one's internal experience, and then make decisions about posture based on bodily cued guidance (rather than following instructions). This approach fosters self-connection and -empowerment, based on the consistent entrainment of somatic self-regulation.

The InnerView principle of attunement addresses the capacity of clients to recover split-off aspects of themselves, given the steady, unwavering gaze of a healer on the person's soul strength. At some point over the course of a two- or three-month series of yoga sessions, someone in the class will come to a point where they want to see me after class. Something triggered her and she wants to process it. As a yoga therapist, while I hear the client's words and concerns, it becomes another opportunity to attune to her nervous system, as well as her awareness of and connection to her own physiology. I offer yoga practices to bring her back into alignment with herself, back to a felt sense of wholeness with her physical experience of the present moment, where she is again empowered to fully feel and choose for herself.

Deborah McDermott has been a yoga teacher for 20 years in the New York City area and is trained in Trauma Center Trauma Sensitive Yoga (TCTSY). She uses yogic techniques to develop felt sense skills, integrating trauma-informed approaches, Yoga Nidra, and polyvagal theory in working with the nervous system. Deb believes empathy is the foundation of connection and healing and incorporates nonviolent communication skills in her practice.

Conclusion

Although the principles of InnerView Guidance were developed for training and supervision purposes, InnerView is also a way to relate to people, and not just to enhance the practices of helping professionals. It comes naturally to young children, whose openhearted gaze conveys curiosity about who you are, not what you do or what you would like people to think of you. It can also be experienced with the elderly when they have not been embittered by life's disappointments. By the time one reaches old age, there are many reasons to be cynical about people and one reason not to be. We are not here to see through people, but to see people through.

The InnerView model offers guidelines for seeing people through their life challenges. These have been presented in the preceding chapters as aspects of an approach based on principles rather than protocols. This means that any helping professional ascribing to one or more of numerous clinical theories and having adopted methods that are a good fit for their practice, can still benefit from the overview that InnerView provides.

The main features of the InnerView approach covered in this book can be summarized as follows:

- To see the person behind the problem.
- To re-envision life situations as soul journeys.
- To work from the innermost self, outward to one's roles in the world.
- To attune to the essence of a person with positive unconditional regard.

We have emphasized the importance of relating to the whole person, by exploring the larger, more meaningful context in which life situations take place and delving into the deeper connections people can make. Both of those must include spirituality if we are to be truly inclusive of the breadth and depth of human nature. In his comprehensive book entitled *Spiritually Integrated Psychotherapy*, Kenneth I. Pargament proposes four main reasons why spirituality needs to take its rightful place in psychotherapy (Pargament, 2007).

- Spiritually integrated therapy is based on the premise that a sense of the sacred has always been a primary attribute of human nature and is a major positive force in the lives of many people.
- Spirituality is a natural and normal part of life whether expressed in healthy ways or not. It represents the quest for the transcendent and the deeply human desire to experience something of ultimate value.
- Spirituality is fully woven into human experience and is part of the therapeutic process whether we attend to it as such or not.
- Spirituality is just as important as medical history, social relationships, and the range of resources for client well-being which need to be taken under consideration for the overall effectiveness of the therapeutic relationship.

What Pargament calls spiritually integrated psychotherapy has long been known by the simple term, soul work. In InnerView terms, it is about understanding what the soul wants and then seeking congruency between the truth of one's inner life and how it is expressed in the world. It is also about the capacity to answer the call beyond ourselves. That will be unique to an individual's path, yet always has universal aspects making it a collective effort whenever we do our part. It keeps us connected with community, since we are profoundly interrelated on the soul level. This is not about private soul-searching for individual enlightenment. It is just the opposite when the elusive happiness we seek comes from gaining skills for self-giving. In the words of Tom Francoeur: "We can't learn skills apart from knowing persons" (personal communication). By knowing persons, Francoeur meant connecting with their essence.

A story told to one of the authors demonstrates a way to relate to "the person behind the problem". One afternoon at Shantivanam Ashram in India, an obviously troubled individual intruded on the peace of the monks and visitors. He threatened them and they felt it was a dangerous situation. Someone ran to find Father Bede Griffiths, a Benedictine monk and leader of the ashram. Upon arriving, Bede faced the man with the steady unconditional gaze we call attunement. Though Bede said nothing, the man began sobbing with the relief of being truly seen. He was consoled and subsequently received mental health support.

As well as having the benefit of our own experiences, we have learned from those who are not professional helpers themselves yet are drawn to InnerView as a path of personal growth. A college professor recently shared her perspective on therapy compared with what she is learning about InnerView. Her firsthand account is a good example of the professional crossroads where we find ourselves, with psychological and spiritual healing still divergent directions for many people.

> I spent six years in Jungian analysis. . . . I found it a very interesting intellectual, moral, emotional exercise. But in the end, though the experience made me wiser about my life, my choices, and my motivations . . . it also made me less happy. . . . With analysis I acquired a sort of seriousness and excessive responsibility that didn't necessarily add positively to my life, if that makes any sense. I began Zen meditation after that, because I felt I needed silence, a clean slate, greater simplicity and immediacy. Although I am quite aware of the benefits, I have become a little wary of therapy or counselling as a result. Considering how a therapy encounter normally works, when I began learning how InnerView differs from the traditional model, it suddenly dawned on me how revolutionary and ambitious it is.
>
> (personal communication)

One of the challenges we face in researching and teaching this model is the need for a new language to discuss the dynamics of soul growth. The language of psychodynamics was formulated in the last century. This has shaped the way some practitioners focus on the pathological aspects of growth and development. Now we need a new language to help us explore what the soul wants and how that can be discerned. Formerly, most soul talk belonged exclusively to religion. We need to find terms that are accessible to the new generation of helping professionals, who are open to the spiritual dimension yet without necessarily having any formal religious identification.

An understanding of spirituality has made inroads in being considered an important part of medical training. It has gained ground with established bodies such as the Royal College of Psychiatrists (RCP) in the UK. Their recommendations for psychiatrists on spirituality and religion concludes: "Given the evidence base, the clinical relevance and the ethical implications, an understanding of religion and spirituality and their relationship to the diagnosis, aetiology and treatment of psychiatric disorders should be considered as essential components of both psychiatric training and continuing professional development" (Cook, 2013).

The RCP website also includes a bibliography of helpful resources for those interested in learning how to assess spiritual and religious beliefs in clinical practice (www.rcpsych.ac.uk/mental-health/treatments-and-wellbeing/spirituality-and-mental-health). One simple tool is the FAITH questionnaire. The letters of the mnemonic stand for *faith* and spiritual beliefs (including questions on what gives life meaning), *application* of faith in daily life, *importance* of faith or belief when faced with illness or health care decisions, the role of faith in *terminal* care decisions, and the need for the kind of *help* provided by a spiritual counsellor or advisor (Neely & Minford, 2009).

Helping professionals who would like to explore the convergence of psychology and spirituality with us further, or who would like to arrange a personal or professional consultation are invited to contact us through the InnerView Guidance website: www.innerviewguidance.com

Ever since Socrates said, "Know thyself" and Shakespeare wrote, "To thine own self be true" there has been the path and practice of InnerView. We have given it a name and some guideposts along the way. We look forward to hearing from our readers and learning more with you, from your own experiences of soul growth to get a sense of the potential for our research, teaching, and consultations. We hope that along with an understanding of the InnerView principles presented in this book, we have renewed the sense of adventure that comes with charting new territory. There is much landscape left to be explored on this journey towards the synthesis of psychology and spirituality which we sum up as soul work.

References

Cook, C. C. H. (2013). *Recommendations for psychiatrists on spirituality and religion.* Royal College of Psychiatrists Position Paper PS03/2013. London: RCP.

Neely, D., & Minford, E. (2009). FAITH: Spiritual history-taking made easy. *Clinical Teacher, 6*, 181–185. https://doi.org/10.1111/j.1743-498X.2009.00317.x

Pargament, K. L. (2007). *Spiritually integrated psychotherapy: Understanding and addressing the sacred.* New York, NY: Guilford.

Further Reading

The reader is encouraged to explore this selected bibliography for psychospiritual perspectives which can be applied to the helping professions.

Almaas, A. H. (2004). *The inner journey home: Soul's realization of the unity of reality*. Boston, MA: Shambhala.

Andrews, L. M. (1989). *To thine own self be true: The relationship between spiritual values and emotional health*. New York, NY: Doubleday.

Bly, R. (1995). *News of the universe: Poems of twofold consciousness*. San Francisco, CA: Sierra Club.

Brooks, D. (2015). *The road to character*. New York, NY: Random House.

Campbell, J., & Moyers, B. (1988). *The power of myth*. New York, NY: Anchor.

Christou, E. (2007). *The logos of the soul*. Putnam, CT: Spring.

Corbett, L. (2015). *Sacred Cauldron: Psychotherapy as a spiritual practice*. Asheville, NC: Chiron Publications.

Culliford, L. (2011). *The psychology of spirituality: An introduction*. London: Jessica Kingsley Publishers.

Frankl, V. E. (2000). *Man's search for ultimate meaning*. New York, NY: Perseus.

Hillesum, E., & Hoffman, E. (1996). *Etty Hillesum: An interrupted life and letters from Westerbork*. New York, NY: Henry Holt.

Hillman, J. (1992). *Re-visioning psychology*. New York, NY: Harper Perennial.

Hillman, J. (1994). *Insearch: Psychology and religion*. Putnam, CT: Spring.

Hillman, J. (1997). *The soul's code: In search of character and calling*. New York, NY: Warner Books.

Hollis, J. (2010). *What matters most: Living a more considered life*. New York, NY: Gotham.

Khan, P. V. I. (2000). *Awakening: A Sufi experience*. New York, NY: Tarcher/Putnam.

Kopp, S. B. (1982). *If you meet the Buddha on the road, kill him! The pilgrimage of psychotherapy patients*. New York, NY: Bantam.

Kornfield, J. (1993). *A path with heart: A guide through the perils and promises of spiritual life*. New York, NY: Bantam.

Moore, T. (1988). *Care of the soul: How to add depth and meaning to your everyday life*. London: Piatkus.

Muller, M. (1992). *Legacy of the heart: The spiritual advantages of a painful childhood*. Palmer, AK: Fireside.

O'Donohue, J. (2004). *Anam ċara: A book of Celtic wisdom.* New York, NY: Harper Perennial

O'Hanlon, W. (2015). *Solution-oriented spirituality: Connection, wholeness, and possibility for therapist and client.* New York, NY: Norton.

Pargament, K. I. (2011). *Spiritually integrated psychotherapy: Understanding and addressing the sacred.* New York, NY: Guildford.

Peck, M. S. (1978). *The road less traveled: A new psychology of love, traditional values, and spiritual growth.* New York, NY: Touchstone.

Richo, D. (1991). *How to be an adult: A handbook on psychological and spiritual integration.* Mahwah, NJ: Paulist Press.

Rieff, P. (1987). *The triumph of the therapeutic: Uses of faith after Freud.* Chicago, IL: University of Chicago Press.

Rosenberg, M. B. (2003). *Nonviolent communication: A language of life* (2nd ed.). Encinitas, CA: PuddleDancer.

Stern, K., & Joseph, M. (1955). *The third revolution: A study of psychiatry & religion.* San Diego, CA: Harcourt Brace.

Vieten, C., & Scammell, S. (2015). *Spiritual and religious competencies in clinical practice: Guidelines for psychotherapists and mental health professionals.* Oakland, CA: New Harbinger Publications, Inc.

Watts, A. (1975). *Psychotherapy east and west.* New York, NY: Vantage Books.

Welwood, J. (2002). *Toward a psychology of awakening: Buddhism, psychotherapy, and the path of personal and spiritual transformation.* Boston, MA: Shambhala.

Williams, H. A. (1992). *Tensions: Necessary conflicts in life and love.* Springfield, IL: Templegate.

Index

3 20